Choosing Health

A One-Size-Doesn't-Fit-All Guide to Diet, Exercise & Motivation

By

Rebecca Hazelton

www.ChoosingHealthNow.com

Publishing services provided by

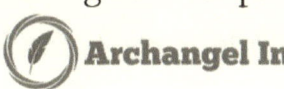 Archangel Ink

ISBN: 1517326648

ISBN-13: 978-1517326647

For Beren, my brother and lifelong inspiration.

Special Thanks

My husband Rylan for ongoing technical support and general wonderfulness.

My sister Jessica for graphic design expertise and moral support.

Erik Schmidt, Kelly Bixler and Nicole Huber for their editorial work and enthusiasm for this project.

Thank you to all of my family, friends, clients and community for helping this dream become a reality.

Content

Foreword

Not the Atkins Diet. Not the Pritikin Diet. Not the South Beach Diet. No "one" diet is right for everybody. Nor is there one exercise program that is right for everybody. In fact, no health program of any sort can accurately claim to be right for everybody. There is something else going on that modern health and fitness care does not account for.

We see examples of this generic approach every day in our workplace, our homes, schools and communities. We observe supposedly brilliant and well-educated people struggling with poor health while they try every kind of diet and exercise program available. Others seem to be fit and healthy with little effort. It was only a matter of time until we started to ask ourselves why.

The answer almost inevitably has to do with this concept called biochemical individuality. Rebecca is very well versed in this subject and, in her new book, demonstrates how Metabolic Typing® can identify the elements that make us different from one another. While it is difficult for some people to grasp, learning one's Metabolic Type is clearly the missing link in every other nutrition program, and a key reason why so many people fail to reach the goals they have for their bodies and for how they feel about health in general.

However, even when armed with this extraordinary knowledge, some people still fail to get and stay in good shape. There is another missing ingredient in most programs designed to help one improve his or her health and fitness. The truth is, many people just don't believe anything will work for them. They have self-limiting beliefs and emotional attachments to being out of shape.

Rebecca Hazelton has brought together both amazing technology, such as Metabolic Typing®, and a unique brand of self- help methodology designed to conquer fear, self-doubt, negative beliefs, procrastination and sheer mental laziness. Her many years experience with personal training and motivation combined with the study and practice of nutrition and individual metabolic requirements has allowed her to bridge the gap between knowing what to do and being able to do it. Choosing Health paints a clear roadmap that anyone can follow to achieve better health. Rebecca's strategies for motivation put the reader into the right mindset to use her guidelines to make some profound life changes.

So, whether you are in good shape and just want to maintain it, or if you are starting from scratch, this book can drastically change the way you make and keep commitments to your personal health journey. The results you achieve may exceed your greatest expectations.

Reed Davis, CMTA, FDN
Founder of Functional Diagnostic Nutrition®

Introduction

I wrote this book for many reasons. While my professional reasons are strong, my personal driving force for writing this book—and for becoming a nutritionist in the first place—is even stronger.

In April 2001, my younger and only brother, Beren, was diagnosed with cancer at the age of eighteen. After a little over a year and multiple rounds of chemotherapy, the cancer continued to spread and the doctor visits that started out enthusiastic with "many options" became quiet with lots of "we could try such-and-such, but..." Beren decided that he would not like to receive any more chemotherapy. This was hard for all of us to hear even though the chemotherapy was no longer helping him.

On July 16, 2002, at seven o'clock in the evening, surrounded by his friends and family, he died.

It was less than six months later that I had "the dream"—a dream that literally changed my life. In this dream my brother was young, maybe four or five, and I was an adult. There were other things happening in the background of the dream that I do not remember, but the part that was significant I will never forget. He reached out to me with something in his hand: a bright red tomato.

It is important to know that at that point in my life, I had been considering going back to school for nutrition. I had pretty much talked myself out of it for various reasons: it would be too hard, too much work, too time consuming, too expensive, etc. In spite of all the "toos," a part of me still very much craved that knowledge. I had been doing a great job of suppressing that desire. Until the dream.

Until the knowing half-smile and look in his eye as he cocked his head to the right and reached out his hand to give me that bright red tomato.

Even in the dream, I knew that there was some deeper meaning. The exact meaning wasn't clear, but I walked closer and accepted the tomato from him. I knelt down and put an arm around his waist and started telling him about the phytonutrient lycopene in tomatoes and how it is important for our health. I awoke shortly after and the dream was swirling in my mind. I quickly jotted it down and then went about getting ready for work. I couldn't tell you the exact moment that the full realization occurred, but when it did, it was undeniable: I was going to become a nutritionist, and all the fears and arguments about how much work, time, etc., no longer mattered. I realized that life is too short to put off those things that we were meant to do, things that give us meaning and a deep sense of accomplishment. Personally, that meaning brought with it the desire to help people with their health.

For me, it took a love that I can only describe as a love that a parent feels for his or her child to give me the strength and conviction to dedicate my life to helping others learn to eat healthier and take better care of themselves. I can teach through example the importance of pushing past fear to get to a place in life that you feel you are happy with yourself and proud of who you've become. If Choosing Health helps even one person to become healthier and commit to making improved dietary and exercise choices, then my dream is realized.

Preface

Over the years, I have worked with hundreds of clients through countless struggles as well as successes. It didn't take long to see patterns emerge. Many people had common obstacles, yet the same solution did not work for everyone. As I experimented with different tactics and tailored my style to fit the needs of each very different client, I learned to become better at helping people through their health challenges. I learned to appreciate people's unique struggles when it came to getting healthier and realized that many of us can initiate change with the right set of tools and the right support.

If you want to change your health for the better but don't know where to start, this book is for you. If you are busy, stressed, or overwhelmed by the magnitude of health tips, diets, and fitness crazes, this book is for you. If you are sick of trying to change your health and failing time and time again, this book is definitely for you!

Choosing Health is designed to give motivation and focus for those of you who struggle to achieve a healthier lifestyle. The greatest gift we have is our health. So many people take it for granted every day, hoping to magically avoid disease and illness because they feel they are too busy, too overworked, or too weak-willed to make any significant changes. I understand that change is hard, but you must ask yourself: Do you really want your life and your health to be left to fate? For those of you who don't want to go another day leaving your health and well-being to chance (and will at least entertain the possibility of giving up the excuses), Choosing Health will give you the tools to make health a conscious choice.

Choosing Health will give you the information you need to make attaining and maintaining a healthier lifestyle possible. Away with the one-size-fits-all approach that is supposed to work for everyone but doesn't! You will learn how exercise, proper diet, and the right attitude are the key elements of a healthier lifestyle. You will be guided every step of the way and will learn how to take care of yourself and your health. You will learn to believe in yourself and your ability to make healthy choices.

Before you begin this exciting journey, take a deep breath.

Breathe in. Let it out fully. And thank yourself for taking the first step toward a healthier you.

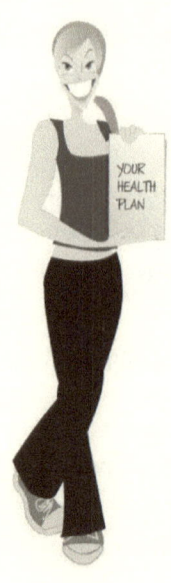

Section 1 Getting Started: Why Should I?

Chapter 1

Hello Health, Goodbye Fear

WHO AM I?

Health isn't only for genetically blessed hard-bodies. Anyone can be healthy with the right attitude and approach. Before we get started, let me ask you something. Can you imagine yourself as healthy?

WHAT IS HEALTHY?

For all intents and purposes, I am defining the holy grail of "health" as a state of being in which you are vibrant, energetic, able to participate in physical activities that you enjoy, mentally and emotionally content, and free of debilitating disease. If you don't fit this description right now, don't worry. You can get there. First things first: you must believe it to see it!

GETTING REAL WITH YOURSELF

In order to become a healthier person, you must genuinely identify yourself as someone deserving of health and willing to describe yourself as "a healthy person."

You must lose any labels you or other people have used that describe you in negative terms, such as "fat, junk-food junkie, sugar-addict, lazy" and so on. If you hold onto these labels and your old self-concept, any changes you make to your behavior will not sink in and affect your identity, they will only be things that you do. While behaviors are extremely powerful actions that you can take toward changing yourself, they are not enough to bring about lasting changes unless you also change how you see yourself. Your behaviors must be congruent with your self-concept.

You may not know it, but you have already made some tough choices:

- Do I want to explore the option of getting healthier? Yes, or you would not have bought this book and you would not be reading it now.
- Do I think this book can help me? Yes, at least some part of you has faith that you can improve your health with proper guidance.

I've always been better at things when I had some confidence in myself. Only you know how much confidence you have in yourself regarding your health. That confidence depends a lot on your life experience up until this point. Do me a favor and answer a couple of questions:

- What is the number one reason you are reading this book?
- If you could reach only one health goal, what would it be?
- What will be your biggest challenge to reaching your health goal(s)?

By the time you finish this book, you will have accomplished at least two things that some people never will: stating a goal that has life or death consequences and admitting a weakness that you had to overcome before you had a chance at long-term success. Sound scary? It is a little. It's also incredibly exciting and empowering!

We let fear prevent us from doing a lot of things that would otherwise allow us to live more meaningful lives. When it comes to our health, we really can't afford to ignore our action-stopping fears. We have to acknowledge them and try to work through them.

We each have a style of approaching things we'd rather avoid. For those of you who have no clue how to face your health-related fears, let me help by giving you some common obstacles and some examples of how one might go about working through them:

- I have no idea how to change.
- What if I reach my goals and I'm still not happy?
- I've failed before and can't bear to fail again.
- If I can't lose weight, no one will love me.
- I can't make the commitment to myself.

Be honest—have you thought any of these before? All of them?

If you have, don't feel bad. Even the most successful health remodeler has had doubts. Learning how to do the work to face these intimidating challenges (and then actually working through the challenges) is how you become the person you can be proud of.

WHAT DO I WANT TO CHANGE?

Let's start with the first obstacle: "I have no idea how to change." One way to approach this obstacle is to define what it is you would like to modify. Once you know exactly what you want to change, it is much easier to explore how you can accomplish it. Write down your answer or talk to a friend about it. When you have a clear idea of the "what," then it is time to work on the "how"—and that is why you are reading this book! By the time you are done, you will know exactly how to make improvements. Obstacle number one solved.

I THINK, THEREFORE I AM... HAPPY?

"What if I reach my goals and I'm still not happy?" This is something we should clear up right away. Reaching your goals does not mean that you will automatically be happy if you are not happy already. Happiness is a state of mind, not a circumstance. Some people have a much easier time finding this state than others. Some people unknowingly give up control over their own emotional state and allow it to be easily influenced by their environment. I'm not saying that if you lose your happy feeling when your boss yells at you or if you get a flat tire, you are weak or emotionally under-developed. I'm not saying that at all. However, the fact remains that you can choose how long you let your mood be affected by things you cannot control. You have the ability to be in charge of your emotions. You have the power right now to be happy. What you may be missing is the know-how.

A LESSON IN EMPOWERMENT

I learned how very able I was to control my mood (regardless of what my environment threw at me) my senior year in college. I was taking a class with Dr. Frank Andrews called Personal Empowerment and he gave the entire class an assignment. I'll never forget it. He told us at the end of class that our assignment for the week was to "have a great day." Literally. We had to decide before the chosen day had begun which day was to be our "great day" and follow through. Jaws dropped, students snickered, and others had looks of either confusion or fear. Regardless of our reaction to the assignment, there it was and we all had to do it.

Being the anti-procrastinator that I am, I decided right away that I would have my "great day" the very next day. The day started out "great" enough, but then my environment made me perfectly aware that it wasn't going to be easy for me. All sorts of things started to go "not-so-great." Extra homework, a hard day at work, an argument with a friend, etc. With each of these hurdles, it would have been easy to say "Forget it! Today sucks and I will try again tomorrow." And I could have done that . . . but I didn't. I talked myself through each obstacle, determined to have my great day. Guess what? It worked!

The power of the mind is amazing. If you set your mind on being happy, you will be. You will find a way. Reaching your goals will just be the icing on the cake. (There really should be a healthier analogy here...the balsamic on the salad perhaps?). Once you build a foundation for yourself in which you believe in your ability to control your emotional state, all of the successes to follow, while rewarding, are secondary.

IF AT FIRST YOU DON'T SUCCEED, TRY IT AGAIN WITH A BETTER PLAN

"I've failed before and can't bear to fail again."

Failing is a harsh way of saying that things didn't work out as you planned. It can be really disappointing when things don't work out how we want them to...BUT, and I know it sounds cliché, if you never go after the things you really want, you definitely won't get them and you won't be living your life the way you truly want. What kind of life is that?!

Instead of being so afraid of trying and failing, I suggest taking smaller, well-thought-out steps toward what you want. This will decrease your chances of things "not working out as you planned" and give you the opportunity of building your self-esteem back up so that you have more confidence in your efforts. For example, if you have a dream to run a marathon, start by walking to the end of the block three days per week. It may not sound like much, but even a small step such as that can have a large impact on regaining trust and confidence in yourself.

The other thing you should consider is whether you are setting yourself up for failure by setting unrealistic expectations. Try to give yourself a generous amount of time to achieve results and set a small goal toward your larger goal. Once you reach your small goal, reassess how you feel before moving forward. If you move forward and you are feeling exhausted and unmotivated, the timing is not right or maybe it is time to change your approach for reaching your goal. By giving yourself a moment to reflect, you can save yourself a potential meltdown and feeling like you failed yet again. Using the same marathon example, you could sign up for a short race first and give yourself plenty of time to prepare for it. If your experience with the short race is unpleasant, reassess your original goal. Maybe you'll realize that you're going to need more time to train than you originally thought.

Give yourself permission to take as much time as you need to reach your long-term goal as long as you continue to make small steps in the direction that makes you feel that you are fulfilling your work toward better health.

THINKING GRAY IS OKAY

"If I can't lose weight, no one will love me."

This is simply not true. Black-and-white (all-or-nothing) thinking is a dangerous mind game. If you honestly think that your friends' and family's love for you is dependent on how much you weigh, you are selling both yourself and them short. Another way that you can look at this pitfall is to remind yourself that the people in your life care about you and want you around. The healthier you are, the chances of you being alive for a long time are increased. Besides, when you are healthy, you feel better about yourself and the choices you are making. People like to be around someone who isn't beating themselves up or sabotaging themselves. So, if you are picking up on a weird energy when you are around people, check in with yourself and see if you are falling prey to a self-sabotaging pattern.

If you are, give yourself some affirmations (see Chapter 2) and remember that rejection begets rejection. If you reject yourself, you give others an open invitation to do the same thing. Set a precedent for how you want to be treated and make sure you abide by the same standard.

Getting Committed

"I can't make the commitment to myself."

I think the best reason to get healthy is for yourself. If you feel you

13

can't, it is an indication that you don't think you're worth it. If you don't think you're worth it, you have some work cut out for you.

You will never succeed, no matter how fabulous of a plan you have, if you don't believe in yourself (the following chapter helps you begin to tackle this dilemma step by step).

While you are strengthening your self-esteem, it may help to pick someone to help hold you accountable to becoming healthier. This has to be someone that you absolutely respect and will honor such a strong commitment. You don't want any reason to fall back on this commitment, so don't choose someone who is likely to let you down by not taking it seriously and give you an excuse to fall back into old habits.

I have listed only some of the many health-related fears that our brains can come up with. You are creative and your brain can invent plenty of obstacles to your success. To ensure that you can overcome future fears and roadblocks, you need to understand a lot more about motivation. The following chapter on motivation delves into how you can achieve what is most important to you.

CHOOSING TO NOT LET FEAR CONTROL YOU

Now is the time to choose your level of commitment before moving on to the next chapter. Below are three different goal options in order of increasing commitment. Choose which goal you can commit to at this point in your health makeover. By placing your initials next to your goal, you are deepening your commitment to this positive change AND improving your accountability. After all, none of us likes to be lied to!

CHOOSING TO CHANGE

Please remember any of the goals to which you are committing:

1. I am choosing to redefine myself as a healthy person. I choose to

reread this chapter and visualize each health-obstacle solution happening to me.

2. I am choosing to redefine myself as a healthy person. I choose to spend one week practicing these health-obstacle solutions each time I encounter a health obstacle.

3. I am choosing to redefine myself as a healthy person. I choose to focus on my strengths and not let fear control my life or hinder my becoming a healthier person from this moment forth.

Chapter 2

Exploring Motivation

S uccess is a moving target: You have to keep applying yourself or it will move on without you.

Sometimes it seems as though we have an abundance of drive and can accomplish anything, while other times it seems like the simplest of things are impossible. If you, like so many others, have battled with yourself to get something done, you aren't weak -- you are human. It is common to start out feeling like nothing will get in your way when you set your mind to something, and a week later feel that you must have been crazy to take on such an endeavor. The million-dollar question is: How do we stay in control of this magical switch? The answer lies within us, but we have to know where to find it.

THE QUARTET OF MOTIVATION

To have any hope of mastering our own motivation, we must understand how it works. I have broken motivation up into four parts: a complex array of thoughts, emotions, abilities, and behaviors. Think of each of these components as instruments in a quartet. Each is unique and important and when all of the parts work together, something even greater is created. (I have developed my own theories for this as well as drawing on the brilliant insight of motivational speakers Anthony Robbins and Brian Tracy and psychologists Abraham Maslow and B.F. Skinner.)

Now for those of you who are already feeling yourself getting bored or feel like you are having a school-anxiety flashback, take a deep breath and hang in there. This is the nuts and bolts of understanding the foundation of what makes you tick. So, going back to the four parts of motivation, it isn't enough to know what the components are; we also need to understand how the parts work and what techniques we can use so that they work to our advantage. It is these techniques that you will learn to master by the end of this chapter that will give you the tools and confidence to make change happen.

I. THOUGHTS

I've often said that people who can control their own thoughts have the most potential for success. Learning that you are in control of your thoughts rather than your thoughts being in control of you is the first step in being motivated and successful. Thoughts are just another way of communicating. Instead of using spoken words to talk to ourselves, we use thoughts. This is why you may have heard people refer to it as "self-talk." Though it may not always feel like it, our internal self-talk is controllable. We can choose to think about things once or over and over again; we can choose to think about the good side of things, or we can choose to think about the bad side of things.

A big obstacle we face when it comes to reaching health goals is that most of us do not use self-talk to our advantage. Instead, we get into a rut of negative thinking and let it control us. The truth is that we can stop negative thinking whenever we want. We are able to give ourselves positive reinforcement whenever we need. Whether we do or not depends on us. You will strengthen your control over self-talk by practicing these steps.

STEPS FOR MASTERING YOUR SELF-TALK

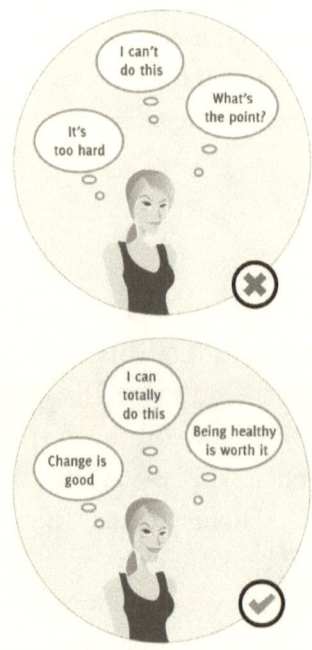

STEP 1: UNDERSTANDING THE CONNECTION BETWEEN THOUGHTS AND EMOTIONS

The first step in self-talk mastery is understanding what thoughts are and how to be in charge of what goes on in your head. Thoughts are really just voices in your head. All these voices in your head are different aspects of you: your memories, your self-doubt, your insecurities, as well as your strengths. Each voice carries with it an emotion and maybe even a persona or character. As we go through life and encounter different situations, the appropriate voice makes comments. These comments are your thoughts.

When repeated enough, the voice is no longer just a voice in your head. It has become a character that is identified by its dominant emotion. Have you ever wondered why our thoughts can carry such an emotional charge? This is how! When we talk to ourselves, we aren't merely thinking. We are feeling a certain way about what we are thinking.

Let me give you an example. When you forget to buy something you really needed at the grocery store, you don't simply think, "I forgot something," do you? No. Your heart beats faster and you get excited, maybe a little angry or frustrated (these are the emotions linked to what you were thinking). Another example; when you do something you think you shouldn't do, do you simply think, "I shouldn't have done that," or do you feel emotions such as guilt, sadness or shame? Our thoughts are strongly linked to emotions.

This overlap of thoughts and emotions is at the crux of why thoughts have such an influence on us. We develop strong associations and they get reinforced over time. Thoughts aren't merely words put together in our heads. They are emotionally charged messages.

STEP 2: IDENTIFYING YOUR CHARACTERS

Sometimes we get so much rehearsal with certain thoughts that it doesn't even feel like we are the ones coming up with them any- more. They seem to develop a mind of their own. It is in this way that our thought patterns develop into "characters." A common example of how we develop thoughts and emotions into characters is that of punishment and parental voices. Some people, whenever they feel like they made a mistake, may hear the voice of their mother or father scolding them. They associate the memory of punishment or shame (emotion) with their interpretation of their behavior (thought). Sound strange? It is, but you probably do it every day and don't realize it.

So, when this association takes place and you feel shame for being scolded by your "parent," stop and think for a moment. Are they in reality scolding you? No! You are creating the internal punishment all on your own. You are the one that assigns the emotion to your thought. You are the one labeling your behavior. Perhaps your parents did scold you when you were a kid, but if you keep repeating that scolding by allowing yourself to think about it every time you make a mistake, you are keeping that association alive. You keep it alive if you continue to repeat it in your head every time something bad happens. By doing so, you perpetuate this cycle of blame and negativity.

STEP 3: THOUGHT STOPPING

Learning to stop thoughts when you need to is a crucial step in the process of mastering self-talk. Negative thoughts cloud thinking and block objectivity, creativity, and healing. You must stop these negative thoughts. There are several techniques. When it comes to thoughts, breaking things down into simple instructions is the most effective and reduces confusion during emotionally stressful circumstances. While it may sound overly simplistic, a tried and true method to changing negative thought patterns is to just say "Stop" when you catch yourself thinking negatively. Don't allow it to continue. If you've allowed negative thinking to happen most of your life, this concept may seem to come out of left field. Believe it or not, you really are the boss of your thoughts. You always have been. What happens when you say "stop" is that you remind your-self of this control. You reinforce that you are the one in charge of the voices in your head. If you apply this simple tool every time (or even most times) that you start thinking negatively, eventually the negative thought patterns WILL stop.

STEP 4: POSITIVE SUBSTITUTIONS

Once the negative thought patterns subside, it is very important to use positive and constructive replacement thoughts to fill the void once filled by all of that negative thinking. You don't want a wide hole hanging around waiting for you to trip and fall into. Now is your chance to be in charge of what thoughts are in your head!

Get out a pen and some paper or type a list of positive reinforcements--things that you can tell yourself to switch your thinking when negative thoughts creep in. Try to come up with a wide variety of positive thoughts that will fit many situations. The more prepared you are, the better you'll be able to put yourself into a positive frame of mind where you can tap into your motivation.

Some examples might be:

"I am ready to accept good things into my life." "I can accomplish my goals."

"I have a strong character."

"Everybody makes mistakes. The important thing is to try my hardest and I will be successful."

"I am a good person."
"We all have our bad days, but I will do my best to make something good happen today."

"I don't compare myself with others. We all have different strengths and I will nurture myself and not belittle my value."

Sticks and Stones

Even though you may follow the directions exactly, negative thoughts may creep in. It's okay, don't beat yourself up. Instead, move on from it and don't dwell. Use some of the affirmations listed above or try some of the following rebuttals to these common self- defeating thoughts:

"I'm too weak."

This is an example of exaggeration. Though it may feel like it sometimes, you are certainly not the only person in the world who struggles with food. Feeling sorry for yourself is your mind's way of trying to get out of facing things that challenge you. It weakens your resolve. Try not to make your situation seem worse than it is. Come up with some examples of other people who struggle with their eating. This will help you realize that you are not in this alone.

Too weak for what? Say specifically for what you think you are too weak. After saying it, do you still honestly believe that you are too weak? If yes, try compromising with yourself and reframe the situation so that you don't feel your overall success is hanging on a single thread. For example: "I am too weak to not eat this cookie" versus "I really want to eat a cookie, but I do not need to eat this cookie right now. I'm going to take a step back from the situation and have some water instead. If I still really want it later, I can eat it and go for a ten-minute walk."

You can also try the affirmation: "The only way to get stronger is with practice. If I start now, I am stronger that much more quickly."

"I'm lazy."

Try to refrain from character-bashing statements like this one. They close the door on all other alternatives and you are left feeling like you are a bad person with no hope of changing. Instead, you can say:

"I am allowed to be lazy sometimes and that doesn't mean I am a lazy person."

Or:

Everyone likes to relax sometimes; that doesn't make me lazy. (Remind yourself of something you did recently that wasn't lazy or of something you can do right now that would make you feel un-lazy.)

"I don't have the self-discipline."

Self-discipline is something few people are born with. Most of us have to work hard to cultivate this virtue. The great thing about self-discipline is that once you practice it several times on easier obstacles, you'll start to see that you do have what it takes to strengthen your resolve. Building self-discipline is much like building a muscle: it takes quite a few repetitions over several weeks before you really feel the difference. Don't quit before you've given yourself a fair shot to improve in this area. You can do it.

"Everyone else except me can eat whatever they want."

This is an exaggeration. Though it may feel like it sometimes, you are certainly not the only person in the world who struggles with food. Feeling sorry for yourself is your mind's way of trying to get out of facing things that challenge you. It weakens your resolve. Try not to make your situation seem worse than it is. Come up with some examples of other people who struggle with their eating. This will help you realize that you are not in this alone.

"I'm a loser."

Again, try to avoid statements like this where all you are doing is beating yourself up. There are about a million different opinions about what makes someone a loser. Do you think that many people are losers? Just yourself? Perhaps looking at others, and yourself, with more compassion will allow you to see yourself in a less judgmental light.

II. EMOTIONS

Understanding how your emotions effect your motivation will help you from getting stuck down the road. It is hard for anyone to reach a goal when they aren't feeling motivated, but if you know how to change your emotional state, you will be able to push through the hard times.

LEARNING HOW TO FEEL

I find it helpful to think about your emotions as feelings that you have learned to have as a result of your environment. Most emotional reactions that we have are socially influenced. For example, some cultures view death as a celebration of life and the entrance into another exciting chapter of afterlife, while some see it as a horrible loss. Neither of them is incorrect and each of them shows how our thoughts affect our emotions. When we enter new territory, our interpretation can get fuzzy and our emotions need more guidance. That is why I am here! Reaching your goals, when all you think you've done in the past is fail, can be new and scary. Sometimes we even go so far as to sabotage our efforts to avoid success because emotionally, we don't know what we're supposed to do.

This sabotage can make us lose sight of our goals. When we lose site of our goals, our thoughts tell us that we should feel upset, disappointed, or any number of related emotions. At this moment, if not sooner, it is crucial for you to metaphorically shake some sense into yourself! Snap yourself out of the emotional hole you are falling into because it is a slippery slope. Your emotions will bend at your will, so you need to take charge of them while it is relatively easy.

Below are some suggestions for taking charge of your emotional state and motivation.

REALITY CHECK

1. Tune into your goal. What made you excited about reaching this particular goal in the first place?

2. Even though you may be frustrated, imagine that you haven't lost any forward momentum and are instead well on your way to achieving your goal. What positive emotions would you feel?

3. Success is like a moving goal post. It's never over. After reaching one achievement, life doesn't just stop. There are lots of exciting adventures ahead of you, so there is no need to get freaked out over reaching a goal. Instead, imagine that life will just go on much the same as it does now with

one big difference: you will feel proud, successful, and healthy! :)

MAKING SENSE OF SELF-SABOTAGE

Sometimes analogies can help ingrain a point which seems too abstract. One way to look at sabotaging thoughts and behaviors is to compare it to being stuck in cement. Since life is all about movement, both physical and otherwise, this analogy is very appropriate. Living your life is about movement and here you are stuck in cement! What is the cement? I define it as any thought or behavioral pattern that keeps you from moving forward, sabotages you, or prevents you from reaching your goals. Using this analogy, think about how often we pour cement on ourselves: We do it any time we do something that disempowers ourselves or contradicts what we strive so hard to achieve. We fall into this cement-pouring pattern by creating an IMPOSSIBLE expectation of success. Take overeating for example. When someone wants to lose weight and they become overweight because they used food for comfort, it is imperative that they stop using food as an emotional crutch. They cannot succeed if they keep overeating, believing that somehow the circumstances will magically change. They won't. The person needs to change. Taking responsibility by accepting that self-talk is the key to change (and using the positive self-talk examples above), will change negative thought patterns that contribute to impossible expectations. This is an important way to stay motivated and be honest with yourself.

WHO'S THE BOSS?

Now it's time to delve deeply into exploring how our emotions can seem so irrational and contradictory. Have you ever wondered why at times we hold two opposing emotional states? Fear and joy when we achieve something? Weakness and strength when we are struggling to make a decision (one side always wins)? One thing is for sure, we are complicated! Mastering our emotional state is a continuous piece of work, but I do hope that my theory of impulse control will help you.

While I am not so sure about Freud's Oedipus Complex, his theory of layers of personality is right on. Even if you only took a basic psychology course in school, you'd have heard of the id, ego and superego. In a nutshell, every person has layers, different aspects of themselves that they present at different times depending on their mood or situation. These aspects of our personalities are not always voluntary. We may not even be conscious of how these different parts of our personality affect our day-to day-decision making, but they certainly do. For example, we have our normal "adult" self that we present to the world at work, social occasions and with our families, but there is another side to ourselves which is much like a child. In a behavioral seminar I once attended, the instructor referred to this child-like self as the id: the part of us that "wants what it wants when it wants it."

YOU ARE ONLY FIGHTING YOURSELF

All of us at one point have seen a child throw a temper tantrum in public. It is not a pretty sight—but it is analogous to how we can act when we want something that we either can't have or know we shouldn't have. Let's use unhealthy food as an example. When our child self wants a food item even though our adult self knows it goes against our health goals, our id fights with us. Our id uses common excuses like "I just want it," "It's not fair that I don't get to have it," or "Everyone else was having some," to get you to cave in. I have heard these very excuses many times when a client is asked about their experience when they gave into a craving. The excuses given are very superficial and irrational and yet they override well thought-out goals with deep emotional importance. Why? Because we don't take charge of our own emotional needs. We aren't listening to our adult selves. We aren't using self-talk to guide us through the irrational "id arguments" that come up every time we want something.

TIME TO GROW UP

It is crucial to your success to understand the adult/id relation- ship and be prepared for the id to rear its ugly head in the moment of decision-making. By understanding the relationship of our adult and child sides, it becomes easier to see through the childish demand.

You can stop telling yourself that you have no willpower. You do. You just need to learn to control it better. Take charge of the id!

The next time you have a craving, visualize yourself in a grocery store with yourself as an adult. Along with you is a child. It can be any child (yourself as a child, even). Now picture the child pointing to the food you are craving and whining that they want it. Then picture yourself as an adult saying no. You can try and rationalize to the child that they can have something else and to not ask for the "bad" food, but this most likely won't work. Let the visualization play out so that the child gets progressively more demanding, screaming and crying and making a scene. Now, you are going to do what I have seen strong parents do: tell the child that the answer is still no and that they can either stay and cry or they can go with you, but that you are done with this tantrum and are turning and walking away. The last step is crucial: visualize yourself walking away. What does the child do once they see that the parent is not going to give in and that their tantrum is futile? They stop and follow you. This is the way to handle food cravings. It works. Our minds are stronger than we think; after all, cravings are just repeated thoughts mixed with emotion. Your "craving" message and your "craving counterargument" both come from the same source—

your thoughts. By understanding that you control those thoughts and by having a technique for handling tough cravings, you will have the ability to control your path in life and persevere through challenging situations.

PRACTICE VISUALIZATION

Visualization is the process of painting a picture in your mind of what you want and imagining yourself getting to that place.

Visualization can be a very powerful tool for helping you overcome roadblocks when you feel stuck. There are many scenarios that you can create for yourself, so practice, explore and see what works for you. Here is one example of an effective visualization exercise that can help you reverse bad habits with good ones by learning to think positive thoughts and not sabotage yourself:

Visualize yourself in a hole, a deep hole. Around you it is cool, damp and dark. If you look up, you can see light at the opening of the hole. Imagine that the only way to get out of the hole is to say positive things to yourself. As you do this, the earth you are standing on at the bottom of this hole thickens and you are closer to the light; closer toward being out of this hole. Each time you say something negative about yourself or to yourself, you dig yourself deeper into the hole.

Now, visualize yourself being happy and successful. What does it look like to you? Feel like? Picture clearly in your mind what your thoughts would be if you weren't saying negative things to yourself. What would you be saying instead? What are some positive things you can say to yourself right now? Say them. Repeat them over and over. As you repeat loving thoughts to yourself, or say them out loud, picture yourself being lifted higher and higher, the hole under you being filled with your positive thoughts. As you come to the top of the hole, warm sunlight washes over your face. Gratitude for life and the powerful influence of your thoughts flows through you. A fragrant breeze enfolds you and as you open your eyes and look around, you see how you are no longer surrounded by dark, clammy walls. You are in the center of a vast pasture with lush grass and wildflowers. It is beautiful and peaceful and you can stay there as long as you like.

Negative thinking will dig you back into the hole. Positive thinking leads you to a place where you have life and beauty surrounding you and your possibilities are endless.

Practice this visualization as often as you need inspiration.

III. ABILITIES

An important step in staying motivated is acknowledging your strengths. Usually, we are all too good at recognizing our weaknesses and we overlook our strengths. Acknowledging both strengths and weaknesses is important for getting a clear picture of yourself.

Depending on your personality, you may be more motivated to excel when you acknowledge your strengths—it makes you feel confident, proud, and ambitious. For others, acknowledging your weaknesses motivates you to take action to become stronger. Which motivates you? One or the other? A combination?

For most of us, being aware of our unique abilities/skills enables us to stay strong and focused. If you don't already know what your unique abilities are, a great way to discover them is to sit down with a blank sheet of paper (or you can do it on the computer) and write a list of five things you think you do well (i.e., communication, hard worker, good memory). Write down whatever comes to mind even if it doesn't seem like an important skill to have. Write it down anyway and try to hold off on judging your list.

Next, list five skills you have developed in your lifetime that you are proud of (these can be anything, i.e., a technical skill, a way of dealing with emotional obstacles, artistic expression, etc.). Lastly, list five things about yourself that you are working to strengthen that you know would make a difference in your self-esteem. Be careful with this last section. This is not an invitation to beat yourself up, but rather an opportunity to strengthen your already powerful arsenal.

I suggested writing five items for all of these writing exercises, but for the first two, you may write as many as you like and have five be a minimum. Even though you may never sit down to write, don't shy away from these exercises. Writing about these topics will really help you learn about yourself—grammar and vocabulary aren't important. You aren't being graded. Spend the most thinking on answering honestly and get down as many thoughts as you can.

Once you've made all of your lists, read through them and add anything you may have left out. This is your template for knowing which strengths can help you on your way to becoming healthier. Add stars to the abilities on your list that might be the most helpful so that you can reference them easily later on if you need to.

While you have some strengths that are unique to you, you also share both strengths and weaknesses with other people. I believe that we are all made up of different amounts of the same ingredients; the same basic construct, but unique at the same time. Some of us, therefore, need more of certain things to flourish in life; some of us may be more sensitive to something than another person. When you have a better understanding of who you are, it helps you to obtain the skills/support that you need to work on the skills that may be holding you back. The exercises you just did in this section will give you confidence as you make lifestyle changes.

It's not till you start climbing to the top and look down at where you started that you realize your capabilities and how far you've come. If you stay at the bottom, your vantage point is always overwhelming.

IV. BEHAVIORS

Power is in the doing! As important as thoughts are in affecting our mood and behavior, there comes a time when you need to stop thinking and act. Don't wait for the right time or for the feeling of motivation to overwhelm you (you may find yourself waiting around for a long time). Take charge right now. Once you do, you will find that at that point, the motivation will follow suit and help you sustain change.

ONLY ONE WAY TO FIND OUT

Behavior is crucial in the process of staying motivated. You've heard the expression, "the proof is in the pudding." This timeless observation reminds us that thinking, feeling and talking will only get you so far: after a certain point, you have to take action. In doing so, you reinforce to yourself that you are capable of more than simply talking about making changes.

What prevents you from taking action? Are you a perfectionist? Do you find yourself revising plan after plan without ever testing it? We've all been victim to the fear of failure before. The truth is that you never know how good or bad a plan is until you try. There is only so much guesswork that you can do. You learn by making mistakes. Only by taking this information and trying again can you ever grow and achieve your goals.

PICKING TOOLS FOR YOUR HEALTH TOOLBELT

As with any stage of motivation, sometimes we get stuck at the behavior stage. Something that worked for us at one point in our lives gets embedded in our minds as a tool to use if a certain situation comes up. The problem lies in using strategies that no longer work.

It is necessary to take a look at your behavioral strategies--your tool belt, if you will--and recycle what no longer works. When you do this, you will notice which habits (behaviors) are still useful and which have become painfully obsolete and hold you back from future success.

Take watching television as a substitute for going out for ice cream. Let's say that years ago, you used to go out to ice cream with your family at the end of the day several times per week and eventually, you developed a weight problem as a result. You decided to take action and instead of going out for the sugary reward, you would instead sit and watch TV with your family. This worked for a while, but pretty soon you found yourself sitting and watching TV every night--whereas before, you went for a walk several nights per week (on the nights you weren't getting ice cream, that is) rather than watching TV. As you can see, the healthy substitution turned out to be only a temporary solution.

WHAT SETS YOU APART?

We learn from our successes as well as our mistakes. Recognition of our behaviors is essential to our success. If you pay attention to what you learn and switch out a behavior that you've learned doesn't work for one that you've learned does work, think of the effect it will have on your confidence. That simple substitution can have more of an impact on your motivation and success than anything else.

THE DEFINITION OF INSANITY

Trying the same thing over and over again and expecting a different result is, by definition, insane! If you turn a blind eye to the information you learn through your experiences, then you're missing the most valuable lesson (and you're insane, to boot). You can't move forward and have a better chance at success if you keep making the same mistake over and over again. When you try something and it doesn't work, think of your brain holding up a big red flag. If you repeat the same mistake, imagine your brain waving the big red flag as if saying, "Hello! You tried this already and it didn't work!" That is your cue to try something else.

DIFFERENT STROKES FOR DIFFERENT FOLKS

One day years ago, my husband and I were making waffles for breakfast and I found that a beautiful metaphor for life was being created before my very eyes. We had the same ingredients: We both had two small waffles, peanut butter, flax seeds, maple syrup, a banana, and a knife. While I spread peanut butter on each waffle and sprinkled flax seed on the peanut butter, stacking the waffles before chopping up the banana and topping with maple syrup—Rylan put banana and syrup on his waffles before stacking them.

This may not sound like it should be that important, but it is a fantastic example of people's unique approaches to life. You can have the same opportunities as someone else and do very different things with those opportunities. This analogy certainly applies to health.

You have, more or less, the same chance at a healthy life as the next person. You make or break that chance with the choices you make and the opportunities you take. Take action when an opportunity presents itself. Don't sit around while others use up all the peanut butter!

CHOOSING HOW TO THINK AND ACT

Now is your opportunity to decide exactly how to change your motivation.

1. I choose to stop negative thoughts the moment I notice that they are sabotaging my motivation or my self-esteem.
2. I choose to write down five things I would really like to accomplish in my life. (Make sure at least one of these things is health-related).
3. I choose to start visualizing every morning what I would be like if I were healthier (how I would look, feel, think, treat others, approach my job, etc.)

.

Chapter 3

Goal Setting

Motivation is useless unless you combine it with action. Goal setting is how motivation becomes more than a hope: it enables you lay out the plan for your goals to become reality. By giving yourself clear, bite-sized pieces of a larger task, the impossible suddenly seems attainable. There are right and wrong ways of setting goals. To be successful, make sure your goals are S-M-A-R-T (ACE Training Manual, p. 377).

S-pecific
M-easurable
A-ttainable
R-elevant
T-ime bound

SPECIFIC

The more specific you are about your goals, the better. Specificity helps you to visualize how your goal will be met. It helps to clarify what it is you really want to achieve. For example, "I want to be healthier," versus "I want to eat at least one serving of vegetables five days each week for the next eight weeks," exemplifies the clarity a specific goal helps us achieve.

MEASURABLE

By making goals measurable, we ensure that when we complete the goal, there will be no question of whether or not we succeeded. With the above example, a food journal could be kept and tallied at the end of each week to know if one serving of vegetables was eaten on five of the seven days.

ATTAINABLE

Attainability is a bit more subjective. Attainable goals are ones that you do not consider too difficult. If your goals are too challenging, you may not reach them OR they will be frustrating to achieve and goal setting will be a negative experience for you.

However, if goals are too easy, there is no real sense of accomplishment when you reach them and therefore not nearly as motivating. Try to choose goals that fall somewhere in the middle of these two extremes and remember that practice makes perfect. Goal setting improves over time and through experience. Setting even small, meaningful daily goals can be very satisfying and will help you perfect the goal-setting process.

RELEVANT

Relevant goals are ones that pertain to your ultimate interest and need. If you want to lose weight, then it would do no good to set a goal, let's say, to read three books per week. While it is wonderful to nurture yourself intellectually, unless the books you read are like this one, setting a goal to read more books is not relevant to a weight loss goal. You'd be better of choosing a goal to start a walking program or choose a bedtime that allows you seven to eight hours of sleep per night.

TIME-BOUND

The last goal criteria, providing a deadline, is essential. Having goals that are time-bound is critical because it keeps you focused and motivated. Deadlines prevent endless procrastination. So many of us put off our goals and don't make them, and therefore ourselves, a priority. You can prevent an aimless goal from being set by giving yourself a time-bound commitment.

KEEPING YOUR WORD

Once you set your goals, the ball toward change starts rolling.

Along the way, you should learn to expect certain things. My hope is that if you are aware of them, you can prepare for them and overcome them rather than letting them push you off course. Making a lifestyle change is extremely difficult. If it weren't, we'd all have exactly what we want in life and we would never struggle; but as we know, that is not how life is. Life is hard and change is part of what makes it hard.

Part of what can help you stay the course of reaching your goals is honoring your commitment. When you make a goal, you are making a commitment to yourself and possibly other people as well.

You will earn respect by following through on your commitment.

You don't want to be the person that says they're going to do something and then never does it, right? No! You want to be the person that when you put your mind to something and say you're going to do it, you keep your word, even though it's hard. That is what builds character. That is what earns self-respect. That is what moves you closer to health.

CHANGING THE WAY, YOU FEEL ABOUT CHANGE

Change can be scary. Change is also what makes you stronger and allows you to become more than what you thought you could be.

You may fear change because you expect it to be hard. There is an alternative way of looking at change that you'll find a lot more motivating. Instead of fearing it, you can instead trust that you can get through change just fine by making small steps (goals) and working at a pace that feels safe to you.

36

It is normal to fear the unknown. Rather than thinking of change as an unknown and possibly unsafe "thing," visualize what it is you want to change. For example, if you want to lose weight but feel that you are afraid and resistant and not really sure why, stop for a minute and think about it. I mean really think about it. Is feeling better about yourself, being healthier, and looking healthy scary? Instead of seeing yourself as someone who can never reach their ideal, see yourself as the person you want to become. Close your eyes and picture it in your mind. Feeling good, feeling strong, feeling in control. Is that what you are afraid of?!

When you really think about it, you'll find, as I have, that we psych ourselves out. Change can be a wonderful thing, especially if it is something that you are in charge of and are setting the road course for how it will happen. Embrace your powerful role in making your life what you want it to be! It is an exciting and wonderful thing.

Don't be afraid; understand it for what it is.

THE CHANGING FACES OF CHANGE

While I strongly believe everything written above, that doesn't mean change always feels like a walk in the park. Sometimes it is downright frustrating. When you feel frustrated, be thankful—this means you are in the second stage of the process. Let me back up. There are three stages of change (depending on which of the many theories of change you choose to believe): honeymoon, frustration, and acceptance (Kirschenbaum, Daniel S).

Stage 1: The Honeymoon

The first phase—the honeymoon phase—is just what it sounds like. People in the honeymoon phase are motivated and excited about their new commitment. They approach their health with zeal and total focus doing everything from measuring out food, to writing down how many calories they burn with each workout. They are so focused on their goals that they think it is easy to take charge of their health. They may even be kicking themselves for taking this long to get on the health bandwagon. For honeymooners, success feels within grasp.

It would be wonderful if we all could just stay in this stage, wouldn't it? But after a month or so (for some it is longer, for some shorter), the abovementioned frustration stage kicks in.

Stage 2: Frustration

The frustration phase is...well, frustrating! Everything that seemed easy before now seems like a huge impossible chore. Even the smallest changes seem too overwhelming.

The goals you set take a backburner and excuses are all too easy to come by. Excuses, in fact, are a big indication that you are in the frustration phase. Excuses reflect that you are not focusing on how to make your goals happen, but are instead looking for a way to let yourself off the hook for not following through with your goals. Sound familiar? For most of us, the answer is yes. This is where most people get stuck. They start out with their goals and move from honeymoon to frustration and then quit. Time goes by and they pick new goals and again move from honeymoon to frustration and then quit again. If that cycle doesn't wreak havoc on your self-esteem, I don't know what does. If you want to learn how to move out of this vicious cycle and out of the frustration phase, keep reading!

Stage 3: Acceptance

Succeeding with your goals and moving into the acceptance phase requires one big thing—commitment! Everything we do, in fact, requires some level of commitment. The more important the task, the more commitment and effort is required...and the more rewarding it is, once achieved. To make it through the stages and into acceptance, first and foremost, you have to accept your fate (and it's not a bad one!). Moving into a stage of acceptance requires that you be congruent with your thoughts and actions no matter what.

No matter how tempting life gets, no matter how tired you are, and whether or not you have the support of others, you commit whole-heartedly to your healthy lifestyle.

PLEDGE OF ACCEPTANCE

To make this point more concrete, I've created the Pledge of Acceptance:

I ACCEPT THAT CHANGE WILL BE HARD, THAT I AM CAPABLE OF IT, AND THAT I CAN DO IT, MUST DO IT AND WILL DO IT.

It is important to really take in these words and commit to what they say. When you are feeling weak and want to give up on your goals, this pledge is what you should repeat to yourself. In fact, repeating it on a daily basis is a great way to affirm your commitment to your health and strengthen your resolve. I guarantee you that there will be times you will want to give up, and will curse yourself forever taking on such an "impossible challenge." But then I hope you will realize you aren't a quitter and that if you give up now, you will come right back to this point again in life and have to start all over! Save yourself the time, energy, and frustration and accept that change gets easier over time and with encouragement. Practice being your own cheerleader and not giving up on yourself when things get difficult. When you prove to yourself that you can follow a goal through to completion, the resulting pride you will feel confirms what you were hoping was true all along: you really could do what you set your mind out to do!

CHOOSING GOALS

Now that we have explored how to properly set goals, it is time for you to practice writing some and learning how to keep commitments to yourself.

1. Say the Pledge of Acceptance out loud to yourself in the mirror.

2. Write down a small goal (one that you can accomplish in a week) using the SMART criteria provided at the beginning of this chapter. Follow through with accomplishing this goal. Make yourself and your goal a priority.

3. Write down a slightly larger goal (one that you can accomplish in two weeks) and tell someone about it. Make yourself and your goal a priority. Once you have reached it, be sure to let that person know!

Section 2 – Nutrition: What a Healthy Diet Should Look Like

Chapter 4

An Overview of the Basics: Eat Well, Exercise, and Set Goals Daily

Most people know that to improve their health they not only have to exercise, but also need to eat well. This simple concept is much harder to achieve than one might think. This chapter is a broad outline into which you can fit all your smaller goals, so that you remember the big picture. When things get confusing and overwhelming, take a step back and take a look at this chapter to remind yourself of what you need to do. Bottom line: pick healthy foods and exercises that you like. You can learn to fine-tune the rest with the suggestions in this chapter.

TAKE YOUR TIME

Some things in this chapter may seem too ambitious for you—don't worry about it. Any of the changes that you make are an improvement to your health. Remember that. I recommend not biting off more than you can chew. Try small changes first and after you can maintain them for thirty days, add in another change.

The biggest mistake you can make and may have already made many times in your previous attempts at becoming healthier, is to try and change everything at once. You may feel like everything you are currently doing is unhealthy, so I can see why you would be tempted to change everything and fully embrace a healthier lifestyle in one fell swoop. However, for most of us, this is too overwhelming and while it may feel great for a short time, chances are that you won't continue for the long haul. That's not to say that that approach never works for anyone; I have seen it work, but it's rare. You know yourself better than anyone else, so choose a pace that you know deep down you can be successful with and stick to it.

Permanent health changes take time and require a period of adjustment each step of the way. You aren't running a race here. There is no finish line. Becoming healthy and maintaining a healthy lifestyle is a process. And the rewards are well worth it.

MAKE YOURSELF A PRIORITY

In order to change, you have to...guess what? Change! For many of us, part of that change includes making ourselves a priority. Say goodbye to the days of putting everyone and everything else before your needs. If you can't put your own health on a pedestal, it'll never get there. It is up to you. Set an example for the cherished people in your life: teaching them to make their health a priority is one of the best lessons they will ever learn.

DEFINING YOUR "DIET"

Traditionally, when someone referred to the word diet, it meant "a pattern of food consumption which is followed by a population or an individual" (retrieved from http://www.answers.com). Diet can also be defined as "...a food regimen designed to promote weight loss in a person or an animal" (http://www.answers.com). Calorie restriction has become so common that I actually have to clarify myself whenever I say the word. Unless stated otherwise, when I refer to the word "diet" from now on, I mean it in the traditional sense of what foods and drinks you consume over time.

LEARN HOW TO EAT HEALTHY

As a nutritionist, I have worked with many people who wanted to lose weight. While there are differences in how each person achieves

43

weight loss, I try to steer people away from quick fixes and drastic changes in their diet. I've said it once and I'll say it a million times: Diets don't work. Their inherent design is to deprive yourself of some type of food, amount of food (or amounts of certain foods), time of day you eat, or a combination of all three for a specified amount of time. Anyone who has ever dieted can tell you, once you stop the diet, you will put the weight back on. It's like magic and it will happen time and time again. This isn't your fault and it isn't a sign that you are weak or a failure; it is a sign that your body is responding accordingly. If you change something in your diet for a short time and then do not continue that change over time, it only makes sense that your body will return to the way it was.

DIETS DON'T WORK

When people diet, they restrict their calories, sometimes to an extreme that isn't healthy. Some diets cut out complete food groups in an attempt to drop pounds quickly. This approach simply does not work for the long run or even in the short run for some people. Are you looking for a quick, temporary weight loss or permanent weight loss? You aren't going to get permanent weight loss from a diet-- period! When you restrict calories and lose weight, about 75% of the weight lost in the first week is water. When you stop the diet, most people go right back to the way they were eating before—the way that made them gain the weight in the first place! It makes perfect sense that if you change the way you eat and you lose weight and don't maintain improved eating habits, your body will respond in kind. How you magically forget this plain and simple fact has to stop or else it will sabotage you! The idea of diets are very tempting and has led to them becoming ingrained in our society. People seem to forget over time how each diet failed to bring them true and lasting weight loss and so they keep repeating the same mistake over and over again. Don't fool yourself or let anyone else fool you into trying the latest fad diet--they simply do not work. What does work is making healthy food choices for your body's unique needs, eating healthy portions, exercising regularly, improving your internal dialogue and setting good goals!

NOT ALL CALORIES ARE CREATED EQUAL

The calories in=calories out theory has led to much of the confusion we have about how to achieve and maintain a healthy weight. Gary Taubes explains it better than anyone (and in EXTREME detail) in his book *Good Calories, Bad Calories*. In a nutshell, our bodies don't treat all calories the same way. There are a plethora of studies that document people losing weight while eating more calories than they previously were. The hormone insulin plays a key role (if you keep your insulin lower, you tend to store less fat) as does biochemical individuality. This biological truth is why some people don't lose weight (or even gain weight on calorie restricted diets). We'll be talking about this much more in later chapters and you will see why eating foods that are right for your metabolic individuality are essential to a happy, healthy body.

WHICH FOODS ARE BAD FOR ME?

Eating right means eating to keep yourself mentally, emotion-ally, and physically balanced. There are so many foods that throw off your blood sugar or jack up your stress hormones, leaving you feeling hyper and then exhausted, cranky, and sluggish. If you eat or drink this way on a daily basis, you probably get colds and flus frequently, have multiple allergies, get headaches/migraines, don't have daily bowel movements or have other digestive problems, have a skin condition such as acne, and lack energy. It will take time to move away from your poor eating habits and towards better choices, but when you do, you will feel and look so much better! The foods and drinks you should make a huge effort to avoid about 99% of the time include:

- Sweetened beverages—Sodas, energy drinks, heavily caffeinated beverages, and juice cocktails.
- Sweets—Candy, most store-bought baked goodies, cookies and cakes containing corn syrup and/or artificial sweeteners.

45

- Low-quality animal products—Meats, milk, eggs, and cheese contaminated with hormones, pesticides and antibiotics. Unfortunately, this is the norm unless otherwise stated on the label (no antibiotics, pesticide-free, no growth hormone, no BGH (bovine growth hormone, etc.).
- Refined and overly-processed foods—Boxed, canned, and frozen foods with added sodium, food coloring, and names on the label that you can't even read. These are all additives that your body doesn't want.

THE GOOD STUFF: WHAT FOODS TO EAT

- Eat whole foods! Eating whole foods, foods that haven't been processed and have come from reputable sources, is your ticket to better health and wellness. Until fairly recently, you would only be able to find these foods at your local health food store or farmer's market, but because of the increased demand, more and more organic and whole foods are available in regular grocery stores. Prices are becoming more competitive every day

- Buy locally and buy organic! Not only do you support local farmers and economies, but the taste and freshness is beyond compare. Buying fruits and veggies locally helps you eat according to what is in season as well, thereby giving your body a variety of tastes and nutrients. Even if there were no nutritional difference between non-organic and organic food, organic food has far fewer harmful chemicals and toxins that your body has to eliminate. These chemicals have known health risks and have no business in your body.

- Be creative! If for some reason you cannot find healthy foods in a store near you and you don't have a farmer's market in your area, there are some great websites from which you can order and have delivered to your doorstep. Many of the distributors for meat/poultry/dairy can be found locally with an online search. Two great United States distributors are U.S. Wellness

Meats (www.uswellnessmeats.com) and Slanker's Grass Fed Meats (www.slankersgrassfedmeats.com). For fruits, veggies and herbs, try your hand at gardening. Depending on time, space, and your degree of a green thumb, you can start a very basic garden (potted tomato plant) or plant different crops year round and actually feed yourself and your family.

The national directory of local farms is eatwild.com. With contact information for 8,000 pasture-based farms, eatwild.com makes it much easier to find quality food no matter where in the United States you live.

A CLOSER LOOK AT ANIMAL PRODUCTS

Dairy

If you're going to consume dairy, I am a huge advocate of raw milk and cheeses. Did a red flag just go up for you? It did for me at first too. I went for years not drinking cow's milk because there was so much controversy about it actually being healthy. After weighing the research, I decided that cow's milk did not seem like a healthy choice and switched to soy milk. I was happy drinking soy milk until someone asked me if I'd heard of raw milk. I hadn't, so I decided to investigate. What I found was such an abundance of credible information on the safety and health benefits of quality raw milk that I couldn't understand why grocery stores would offer anything but raw milk...but then I reminded myself that grocery stores are full of foods and drinks that are harmful to our health!

What Is Raw Milk?

Raw milk is the original milk that everyone used to drink. It is milk that has been taken from the animal (in this case I am referring to cow's milk) and bottled. There is no additional processing.

Growth Hormones

Commercially produced milk almost always contains growth hormone (rBGH, recombinant bovine growth hormone, a genetically modified growth hormone), which is injected into cows after they give birth so that they will continue to produce milk. Cows normally produce milk for twelve weeks. Giving them growth hormones, the farmer can extend the cow's milk production for up to twelve weeks longer. The biggest issues with this practice (and there are plenty) is that rBGH increases the cow's risk of infection by almost 80%, increases the cow's "need" for antibiotic treatment, and increases humans' insulin-like growth factor 1 (IGF-1). In an effort to gain profit, cows are put at a tremendous risk for infection. Even if she doesn't get sick, her body makes milk at the expense of her own tissues, causing her body to be under much stress. I, for one, have no desire to drink milk laden with all those stress hormones. If the cow does succumb to infection, she will be given antibiotics. Those antibiotics will also be passed along in the milk.

Lastly, IGF-1 is a potent growth hormone produced in the human body. As with all of our hormones, balance is key. When we drink cow's milk that is treated with rBGH, our IGH-1 levels can increase by as much as nine times their normal level! Since IGH-1 is a known hormone that regulates and accelerates several types of cancer, there is a huge risk in drinking commercially produced milk that doesn't specifically say on the label "free of rBGH hormone."

Pasteurization and Homogenization

Most milk that you find in the grocery store is processed in two ways: pasteurized and homogenized. Pasteurized milk has been heated to 161 degrees to kill bacteria and extend shelf-life. Sounds good, right? Wrong! Read the excerpt below for a full understanding of what happens to milk once it is pasteurized. If you still want to drink pasteurized milk after knowing what it is, at least you will have made an educated decision. After pasteurization, bacteria found naturally in milk are killed. During the high-temperature heating process, cell bodies of these bacteria are ruptured and their contents are spilled, releasing histamines. This causes many milk drinkers to suffer allergic reactions. Almost all of these same consumers can drink raw milk and not have allergies. The high levels of bacteria permitted in milk intended for pasteurization are still found in pasteurized milk; they are just dead and not removed by the process. (retrieved from http://www.organicpastures.com/faq. html). Yes, that's right. When you drink pasteurized milk and milk products, you are also ingesting a nice dose of ruptured bacteria.

Milk companies should think of changing their "Got Milk?" slogan to "Got Bacteria?" Somehow, I don't think they'd get nearly as many yesses. And don't even get me started on homogenization. That is a whole other can of worms. We trade unadulterated fat molecules from milk (natural molecules that our bodies recognize) for pressure-treated "smooth" milk fat (broken up, blended fatty remains that may contribute to heart disease and arterial plaquing). Am I the only one that sees a problem here? Luckily, no. The Weston A. Price Foundation has quite a bit to say on the matter. I have included one excerpt for your reading pleasure:

Pasteurization destroys enzymes, diminishes vitamin content, denatures fragile milk proteins, destroys vitamins C, B12 and B6, kills beneficial bacteria, promotes pathogens and is associated with allergies, increased tooth decay, colic in infants, growth problems in children, osteoporosis, arthritis, heart disease and cancer. Calves fed pasteurized milk do poorly and many die before maturity.

Raw milk sours naturally but pasteurized milk turns putrid; processors must remove slime and pus from pasteurized milk by a process of centrifugal clarification. (retrieved from http://www.realmilk/what.html). For much more information, please visit http://www.realmilk.com/. You will receive the education of a lifetime.

What Happened to Raw Milk?

In a nutshell, up until 1908, pasteurization was not standard processing for milk. Most people drank raw milk. Sadly, raw milk is becoming more and more difficult to find and is illegal in most states. Ridiculous but true.

People are uneducated and miseducated if they think that commercially produced milk is safer than raw milk. The media paints a favorable picture of commercially processed dairy. They don't tell you that almost every single bacterial contamination in the past one hundred years has been from pasteurized milk, not raw! After reading this chapter, you now know the truth. For a list of where you can find raw milk near you, please visit: http://www.rawmilk.com/where1.html.

I must add that I don't believe adults "need" milk. Water and nourishing foods are ideal. However, if you are going to drink milk, raw is far superior.

Meat

Moving along to other nutritious food choices, if you eat animal protein, I strongly encourage you to buy free-range meats, poultry and wild-caught fish. Toxins such as pesticides, heavy metals, growth hormones and antibiotics accumulate in the fat cells of both humans and animals (http://www.liverdoctor.com/index. php?page=liver-problems&subpage=toxins). These toxins are thought to be the cause of many diseases including cancer and high blood pressure. The nutritional implication of this is that you want to avoid as much of these toxins as possible. To do this, you will want to buy quality animal products. They will have substantially less fat, better quality fats (explained in detail in Chapter 6), and less toxic residue because of their better diet (Fife, 2001).

Grain

If you eat grains, try to eat whole, sprouted grains instead of processed, nutrient-robbed grains (see Chapter 5, Carbohydrates, for specifics). Not only do you get more nutrients when you eat whole grains, but you also have a better chance of avoiding bleach, food colorings, preservatives, and added sugars (Whitney & Rolfes, 2002). The more you stay away from processed foods and get back to basic nutrition, such as combining whole foods, the better you will feel, the less toxins you will absorb, and the more money you will save.

Supplements

I fully support the ideology of getting all of your nutrients through the foods you eat. However, because of poorer soil quality, stress (environmental, chemical, physical, emotional, mental), and chemically treated foods, the reality is that all of us need some additional nutrients to uphold optimal health. When deciding which nutrients to supplement with, I advise that you seek the help of a professional. This will help ensure that you will be taking the right combination for you. A general rule as to the quality of supplements are to choose brands that do not add artificial colors, flavors, or fillers and choose a high potency food-based product to improve absorption and reduce chemical load. Ultra Life (www.ultralifeinc.com), Standard Process (www.standardprocess.com), BioMatrix (www.biomatrixone.com), and Nordic Naturals (www.nordicnaturals.com) are but a few of the reputable supplement companies you can order from.

RELEARNING HOW AND WHEN TO EAT

What to eat is incredibly important, but you also need to know how and when. Eating too quickly is a big no-no. Take your time with your eating and chew your food thoroughly. This sounds so basic and yet every day I see people wolfing down their food and it often isn't because they are in a hurry. We have become out of touch with our eating behavior. It is as if we become hypnotized when we eat and we feed ourselves in a trance.

There are many negative repercussions with this: not enjoying your food fully, overeating and weight gain, not feeling satisfied/satiated, and, not chewing properly can cause digestive distress and poor nutrient absorption. The longer that we go without eating mindfully, the more the "automatic pilot" behavior becomes ingrained in us and the harder it is to change the habit.

Also, for the best digestion, take small sips of water (or do not drink anything) with your meals. Drink water 15-20 minutes before and after you eat so that you do not dilute your digestive juices!

Mindful Eating vs. Bored Eating

Have you ever seen people eating (or been one yourself), and after finishing what is on their plate, they look around, and seeing that others are still eating, decide to go ahead and get seconds so they have something with which to occupy themselves? It is a vicious cycle. Their own hurried eating behavior sets them up for over- consumption of food and calories. If they'd slowed down, they would be in tune with the satiety signals their body was sending, they would have enjoyed their food more and felt more satisfied, and the extra time they would have spent eating slowly would have allowed the other people to finish so that the social pressure/visual cue to eat wouldn't be there. Chew your food and take sips of water in between bites*, set down your fork or spoon and take a deep breath and assess if you are still hungry or if you are continuing to eat simply because the food tastes really good.

I've often come to the point in my meal where I feel full and still have food left on my plate, but it tastes so good that I want to keep eating. This tendency is fairly common. So what can you do? You have two choices: you can keep eating and feel uncomfortably full afterward, consume far more calories than your body can use, and perpetuate the cycle of eating too much in a sitting OR you can remind yourself that the food is going to taste just as good later and push your plate away. Take the rest of it with you and eat it at your next meal when you are actually physically hungry and not just caught up in the moment.

Being too goal-oriented is not a good thing when it comes to finishing a meal. We are so conditioned to feel satisfaction once something is "finished" and not before, and this concept is key when it comes to changing your eating behavior.

You do not need to finish the food on your plate, in your reclosable snack bag, etc. If this does not seem like a concept you can grasp, you need to prepare smaller portions. Before you start eating, make sure your portion is reasonable so that if you do eat it all, you will not be sabotaging your healthy eating habits or your waistline.

Avoiding Plummeting Blood Sugar

To avoid problems with your blood sugar and blood-sugar-regulating hormones, aim to eat every three to require prior planning to make sure that you have food with you for snacking no matter where you are (stuck in traffic, on the bus, in a meeting, on your way to the grocery store, etc.). It is not a good idea to push yourself till you have a headache and are cranky before you sit down to nourish yourself. There is a reason why those symptoms occur: it is the brain's way of telling you that it needs food right now and that you missed its more subtle warning signs.

Your brain and body will function better if you fuel it at regular intervals. Eating on a three-to-four-hour schedule requires that the size of the meal be relatively small. When you eat the right combination of carbs, protein and fats, you will not be inclined to overeat because your body feels satisfied. Aim for around 250-600 calories depending on your height, weight and metabolic type® (*Metabolic Typing® is a testable, repeatable nutrition technology that takes the guesswork out of what each person should eat.) and eat a balanced meal. In general, taller people with a lot of muscle require more calories per day.

Your mini-meal should contain a mix of protein, carbohydrates, and fat. Depending on your unique chemistry, the amounts of protein, carbs, and fats you need at each meal will vary. More on this later.

Many foods fall into more than one category and that makes things easier when you are packing your food for the day. Some examples are a mozzarella cheese stick and a piece of fruit. The cheese has both protein and fat and the fruit is primarily carbohydrate. This method of food combining will leave you feeling more satisfied and will stave off hunger for longer than if you had an all-carbohydrate, all-fat, or all-protein meal. Here is a short list of the many possibilities you can come up with):

REBECCA'S HEALTHY MINI-MEAL SNACK IDEAS

- Hard boiled egg & tomato
- Celery and nut butter
- Wild-caught mackerel or sardines over salad greens
- Carrots and hummus or guacamole
- Apple slices with organic cheese
- Plain yogurt with berries

- Cantaloupe with cottage cheese
- Veggies and cream cheese
- Tuna or salmon on tomato slices
- Sliced organic deli meat with avocado slices
- Olives and 1-2 ounces of chicken breast or thigh
- Tuna in water, organic mayo, lettuce leaves
- Cottage cheese with almonds
- Pickles and Mozzarella stick
- Jicama and guacamole
- Jerky and sliced veggie
- Egg salad lettuce wrap
- Tuna on cucumber slices
- Smoked salmon, cream cheese, cucumber slices
- Sunflower seeds with cottage cheese

MOVE IT OR LOSE IT

Exercising should be part of your daily regimen. Our bodies are designed to move! To deny ourselves of this basic function is a death sentence that begins with gradual loss of strength, function and flexibility. With our vertical posture and over 600 muscles, we have been activity machines for thousands of years. In the last fifty years or so, however, our lifestyles have gotten more and more sedentary. The invention of convenience appliances and services as well as the popularity of computers both at work and at home contribute to our increasing inactivity. Many people spend their days sitting at work and they come home and sit some more in front of a computer or television. As a result, our postures have begun to round forward, muscles atrophy, and back pain is currently one of the most common chronic pain complaints.

Sedentary Lifestyles the Norm

Personally, I have seen things worsen in just the past ten years-- not only for adults but for kids as well. When I was growing up, I absolutely loved playing outside and being active, as did most of the kids I knew. Look around now and you will see how many more overweight, inactive kids there are compared to when you were a kid. Sedentary activities such as video games, playing on the computer, and watching TV are common. As we age, many of us become more and more out of shape. If you have been waiting for a wake-up call as an excuse to get started with movement, here it is! Sedentary lifestyles beget sedentary lifestyles. It's not going to magically change "one of these days." You must find a way to fit activity into your life. Some suggestions are walking, jogging, or running outdoors, riding a bike in or outdoors, dancing, calisthenics, going to a gym or private training facility, rollerblading or rollerskating, gardening, jump roping, marching in place, yoga, martial arts, etc. Pick something that is fun for you and start!

TYPES OF EXERCISE

If you are doing any movement, give yourself a pat on the back. You are on the right track. I am going to teach you how to establish a balanced workout routine so that you can look and feel your best. In this chapter, we will explore different types of exercise that you should add to your movement repertoire. It is best to start out gradually so that you don't overdo it and lose interest. The three main components of exercise for well-balanced health are aerobic, strength training, and flexibility training. Let's take a closer look.

What is Aerobic Exercise?

Aerobic or cardiovascular exercise uses large muscle groups for rhythmic, sustained movement over a period of time. Aerobic exercise gives your heart and lungs a great workout. Over time, your heart and lungs adapt and become better able to deliver blood and oxygen so that they don't have to work as hard. This increased efficiency is one of the great benefits of cardiovascular training and helps us to live longer, healthier lives.

How Much Aerobic Exercise Do I Need?

A good daily goal is thirty minutes for general health and longer if you are wanting to lose weight (keep in mind that increasing the duration slowly is usually best so that you do not overdo it or injure yourself). If you are currently inactive, start at ten minutes a day of just walking. You'll be amazed at how good your body will feel with even a small amount of movement. When you can easily do ten minutes a day, increase to doing ten minutes several times a day OR try doing it all at once. Wear comfortable shoes and clothes that wick the sweat away from your body. Bring water with you, and if you are exercising outside, it is recommended to wear sunblock.

Strength Training

Strength training exercise uses resistance such as body weight, machines, or free weights to strengthen each muscle group. Strength training is important for strong muscles and bones. It is one of the best forms of exercise for body fat loss, so if you have only been doing aerobics and thinking that lifting weights is only for jocks and body builders, think again. Strength training should be part of all of our weekly routines. Good guidelines for strength training are one to two sets of exercises for all the major muscle groups one to three times per week. (See Chapter 12 to learn more and for a sample program.) It is important to alternate muscle groups when you strength train to avoid training the same muscle group two days in a row. Your muscles need a full forty-eight hours to rest and rebuild. If you do not allow them adequate time to recuperate, your risk for getting injured increases and that can be detrimental to your results and motivation.

Balanced Strength

It is important to strengthen the body in a balanced way (i.e., front and back of the legs, not one or the other), so try not to skip muscle groups. We all have our favorite areas that we like to exercise, but don't forget to work all your major muscle groups (upper back, chest, front and back of legs, buttocks, front and back of lower leg, low back and abdominals).

For building muscle, aim lower on repetitions and higher in weight/ difficulty (8-12 repetitions) and for more general strengthening and toning, aim for 12-15 repetitions or even as high as 15-20 reps and choose a weight that is appropriate to fatigue your muscles in each set. A common misunderstanding is that you have to keep the weight light if you want to avoid building large muscles or do hundreds of repetitions to tone. It is important that you challenge the muscles enough to stimulate change. If you choose too light a weight so that after, say, 15 reps you are not "feeling the burn," it is not heavy enough to challenge your muscles and therefore create a stronger, more toned muscle. Make the weight a little heavier so by the end of the set, you are very relieved.

Flexibility and balance means taking all eight of your load-bearing joints through a full range of motion so that you can avoid limited mobility AND putting the body in positions where it can sustain position without falling (more in Chapter 13). It is important to work on this every day! I recommend stretching whenever you think about it. Not only does it feel great, but it prevents stiffness and lack of mobility. A great way to work on balance is to stand on one foot.

You can do this while you are doing other things such as brushing your teeth or hair. Balance is definitely one of those things that suffers over time if you don't work on it. Falling is never fun, but the older we get, the higher the stakes when you take a fall. Don't be a statistic and break your hip: work on that balance!

When Can I Find Time to Exercise?

"Those who think they have not time for bodily exercise will sooner or later have to find time for illness." – Edward Stanley, the Earl of Derby, 1873. Is my point hitting home? Exercise is something that you need to be doing regularly! The rewards far outweigh the costs. Here are some general recommendations for how to fit exercise into your busy life, but remember that any way you fit it in is an accomplishment. If you can come up with a way to include exercise in your life other than the recommendations given here, go for it!

Make Exercise Your Priority

Make exercising a priority and schedule a block of time somewhere in your day every day that you devote to your fitness. For example, many people find that first thing in the morning is best since they get it done and have elevated energy throughout the day. For some people's schedules, mornings are not always possible.

Remember, any time that you can do it is good--just do it!

Schedule mini-workouts throughout the day rather than doing it all in one fell swoop. This sometimes works better, but you must follow through and accumulate exercise throughout the day. If you find that you start off strong and either lose motivation or just get distracted, see if you can do one or two longer workouts earlier on in the day so that you are getting the desired thirty minutes.

Make your day your workout. If you cannot or will not schedule a "workout," see if you can modify activities that you must do so that you get a bit more out of it. Examples can be walking the kids to school (or riding bikes) versus driving them, parking further away at the grocery store, jogging in place while you sort laundry or talk on the phone, stretching at night with your kids, or using them as your strength-training tools (baby bench press anyone?). Use your imagination and I guarantee that you can find ways to get more movement in your life.

Ready... Set... Action!

By this point, you have the know-how to begin or make changes to a workout. Section 3 of this book, Fitness Made Simple, will look at each of these topics in further detail. I know it may sound like a lot, but once you start exercising in small increments, you'll realize that it is completely doable. Your next step is to commit to exercise goals daily and stick to those goals. As previously stated, it is best to ease into exercise and build on it slowly versus going into it full-bore and either getting injured or burned out.

STAY HYDRATED

There are literally hundreds of choices when it comes to deciding on what to drink. Many of the options are not ideal: colas, fruit cocktails, caffeinated drinks, juices with added sugar or high fructose corn syrup, flavored milks, and drinks with food coloring, preservatives and artificial sugars. The list goes on and on for unhealthy beverages, but for healthy drinks that actually provide the body with water and even some nutrients, the list is much shorter.

Your Body Wants Water

- Water is THE BEST drink you can choose for hydrating your body. Water is one of the six basic nutrients needed to survive (proteins, fats, carbohydrates, vitamins, and minerals are the other five). The human body is on average about 72% water (some organs contain more or less: the liver is around 96% water!). Without water, digestion and absorption would not be possible, nor would regulation of body temperature, removal of wastes and toxins, or assimilation of water-soluble vitamins such as vitamin C. It is medically known that as little as a 5% drop in body fluids will cause a 25%-30% loss of energy in the average person. We could live for quite awhile without food, but only days without water. Besides hydration, important minerals such as calcium, magnesium, and potassium are found in water. Because water can also be contaminated with chlorine, toxins, and other impurities, drinking filtered water should be a priority. If plain water is too boring, adding cucumber, lemon, lime, or orange wedges is a great idea...in fact, one needn't stop with citrus fruits. Adding a few frozen berries instead of ice not only adds color and interest, but tastes great too.

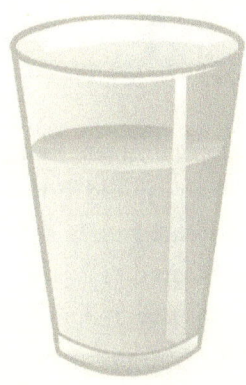

- Carbonated and flavored waters are an okay choice, however, regular, non-carbonated water is best since carbonated water often has added sodium. Make sure to look at the ingredients and avoid added sweeteners, colors, and preservatives. "Essences of fruit" are desirable because they add a bit of flavor without adding calories or sugars.

- Juice that is 100% juice and free of added sugar, corn syrup, fructose, and artificial colors is another healthful choice. Fruit juice is still high in sugar though, so in terms of health and hydration, it is best to dilute juice with filtered water and also drink the freshest, least processed juices available so that you receive the antioxidants and other plant nutrients and enzymes that are naturally occurring and which die shortly after the fruit is juiced.

- Fruit smoothies can be a great summer treat, but beware of serving sizes and ingredients. Keep them as basic as possible (fresh or frozen fruit, ice, a little milk or yogurt of your choice) and around 8 ounces in size.

- Milk can also be a healthful beverage. There are many kinds to choose from: cow, goat, coconut, soy, rice, almond, raw versus pasteurized, organic versus non-organic. As mentioned earlier, they differ greatly in nutritional value. Suffice to say that any of these options are preferable to colas and other highly sweetened, processed, preservative-laden drinks.

- Unsweetened herbal teas are another good option for hydration. Children should not be given caffeine as a general rule and since caffeine acts as a diuretic (encourages the body to lose water), caffeinated teas and other beverages are not ideal for hydration. If sweeteners are needed to make the tea palatable, possible options are stevia, raw honey (not to be used for children under age two), or other natural sweeteners (check with local health food store).

- Coconut juice (not milk) is a great source of electrolytes and helps you stay hydrated.

How Much Water Do We Need?

Now that the answer to the question, "What should I drink to stay hydrated?" has been answered, it is also important to know how much we need to drink to stay hydrated.

First, whether you are drinking tea, juice, or milk, you need to be drinking water! Many of us don't drink nearly enough water each day and suffer greatly for it. In the book, You're Not Sick, You're Thirsty! Batmanghelidj explains in detail just how essential water is. Did you know that chronic dehydration is at the root of many conditions such as high blood pressure, allergies, diabetes, and autoimmune diseases such as rheumatoid arthritis?

A good estimate for how much water you need each day is to take:

Your body weight (in pounds) divided by two. This equals the minimum ounces of water you should drink every day!

For example: a 140-pound woman should drink about seventy ounces of water daily, more if she is active.

This is the minimum amount of water in ounces your body needs each day. If the number seems too high, remember that most people don't get anywhere near the amount of water they need every day.

Headaches, back pain, joint pain, fatigue, moodiness, constipation, thirst, and lack of concentration and coordination can all be signs of dehydration. My suggestion is that you start first thing in the morning and continue throughout the day—don't wait until you feel thirsty because you'll be too late. Our thirst response is delayed, so if you wait until you feel thirsty, you are likely already dehydrated.

To help gradually increase water intake, keep a daily log of how many ounces are consumed (this is easier if you use a container that has the ounces listed on the side). If you notice that you are not taking in nearly enough fluids, don't panic or go on a guzzling fest. Instead, try to increase the amount over time by carrying around water bottles, keeping filtered water at home, avoiding heavily sweetened or salty beverages and foods, and by paying attention to your body's hints that you are thirsty.

REST AND RECOVERY

Sleep is also a critical component to total health. If you are someone who tries to get by on the least amount of sleep possible, STOP IT! You are doing yourself a huge disservice. You may have not been getting enough sleep for so long that you don't even realize anymore how different you feel when you get a full night's sleep.

Your body does a lot of internal repairing as you sleep. Try to get six to eight hours of sleep per night (insomniacs, those with sleep apnea, and parents with newborns, just try to do your best), so that your body can repair itself after a long day. Every ounce of time that you put into your health, even if part of that time is unconscious, is an investment and the payoff is better than anything money can buy.

A Word on Knowing Your Body

I often say that you know your body better than anyone else, but this is only true if you are in tune with your body. Luckily for you, this is a skill you can learn. I started from an early age being told by my father that it was important to eat well and be active and so I am one of the fortunate few that is pretty in tune with my body. I know that if I am feeling cranky, I need to drink water, eat a balanced meal or take a moment for myself. There are millions of people that instead, self-medicate with drugs, alcohol, or medication. There is much to be said for getting back to the basics and getting in tune with your body. Simplify your routine and your diet and take time out to relax even if it's just taking a few deep breaths and reflecting on one positive aspect of your day. These are critical to your health and well-being!

LEARN TO RELAX

I took my first relaxing, tropical vacation when I was twenty-eight years old. I went with my husband and in-laws to Hawaii for nine days. After five days, I noticed how much "lighter" I felt. The day-to- day stresses were left behind and my normal routine and responsibilities had been put on the back burner. Not only did I feel mentally and emotionally refreshed, but my body seemed to have taken a big exhale as well. What a powerful message this feeling was-- that we all need a break sometimes.

I live on a day-to-day basis with a healthy routine. I nourish myself properly, get daily exercise, etc., but there is the important relaxation requirement that I hadn't been getting and probably most of us don't get. Do you allow yourself to relax? I'm sure for some of you, you may feel like you have the opposite problem and are lacking a motivational push. Both are important.

Ways to Relax

There are times to be motivated and there are times when we need to allow ourselves a mental and physical break. This doesn't mean to eat horribly or neglect your body but do it differently than how you do it most of the time. Try some different nutritious foods (and maybe have someone else prepare them for you), do different activities than you normally do (try hiking in a new place, take a healthy picnic), give yourself a chance to reflect on your life—this is something that is so rewarding and so difficult to do when you are in the thick of your daily responsibilities. This "mental vacation" is what so many of us need and so few of us get. How do we give it to ourselves without physically removing ourselves from stressful surroundings or the daily grind without relying on alcohol or drugs? Here are a few suggestions:

- Get a massage
- Relax in a hot tub or sauna
- Go for a hike
- Picnic to a secluded, relaxing spot
- Meditate
- Take a bubble bath
- Read an old favorite book (or just your favorite part)
- Go to the zoo
- Watch a movie

- Listen to some of your favorite music
- Lay out in the sun for a few minutes
- Have some tea
- Stretch or do yoga
- Garden or go sit in a beautiful garden (hopefully your own)
- Do something that you want to do (as opposed to something you need to do)
- Make an "I want" list and put your "to do" list away.

CHOOSING A PLACE TO START

This chapter covered a lot, so don't feel badly if you need to reread it before moving on. All these major concepts will be explained in much greater detail in the following chapters. Now that you know the basics of what a healthy lifestyle takes, where do you want to start first?

1. I acknowledge that I want to be a healthier person and will make small steps toward this transition. I will eat my favorite vegetable at least two times this week and choose a small activity goal (i.e., take a five-minute walk or bike ride, do three strength training exercises at home or at the gym, etc.).

2. I will eat every three hours at least one day this week and observe how I feel differently after my meals. I will reward myself for reaching this goal with one of the suggestions given in the "Rest and Recovery" section of this chapter.

3. I will do both of the above written goals and I will drink a minimum of thirty-two ounces of water each day this week.

METABOLIC TYPING® BASICS

Before moving on to the nutrition section of this book, I strongly urge you to find out your metabolic type®. You can do this in several ways: take the self-test in The Metabolic Typing® Diet (Doubleday, 2000) by William Wolcott and Trish Fahey, available via http://www.amazon.com, or meet with a Certified Metabolic

Typing® Advisor for the Advanced Metabolic Typing® test with on- going guidance and consultation. This is highly recommended!

Contact me directly for consulting or and stay in control of your eating so that you feel satisfied, balanced, and nourished.

The basis for metabolic typing® is that we all have unique biochemistry and therefore unique nutritional needs. Some people do much better when they eat certain foods while others can have the opposite reaction. Metabolic typing® is right in line with the "one-size-doesn't-fit-all" approach of this book.

There are three main metabolic types®: Protein types, Carb types (short for carbohydrate types) and Balanced/Mixed types. These are very broad categories. Actually, there are as many metabolic types® as there are people in the world!

Protein types generally function much better, have more energy and balanced weight when they eat more protein and fat in relation to carbohydrate. Protein types do very well on heavy proteins like red meat and dark meat poultry. Protein types tend to get cranky when they don't eat regular meals and often need to snack between meals.

Carb types generally function better, have more energy and balanced weight when they eat more carbohydrate in relation to protein and fat. Carb types do well on lighter meat poultry, fish, vegetables, whole grains, and relatively low amounts of fat. Carb types tend to forget to eat, fill up easily and often do not need to snack between meals.

Balanced/Mixed types generally function better, have more energy and balanced weight when they eat a balance of protein, fat, and carbohydrate. Balanced/Mixed types can swing to either extreme of appetite if they do not eat the right balance of protein, fat and carbohydrate.

With every single person, no matter what their metabolic type®, it is essential to eat the right amounts of protein, fat and carbohydrate at every meal. Mastering the art of balancing your meals is one of the greatest benefits you will gain when you learn your metabolic type®.

The illustrations of plates of foods below are just three examples of the many possible ratios of protein, fat, and carbohydrate you can eat at each meal. There is a right ratio for you just waiting to be discovered!

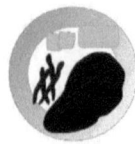 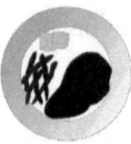 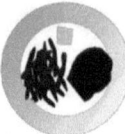

Chapter 5

Carbohydrates

Carbohydrates or "carbs" have gotten a bad rap as of late. Since weight loss can be frustrating, we are quick to find a scapegoat to place our blame. Carbohydrates are not our enemy (nor are any of the other macronutrients, such as protein and fat). Once you understand which carbs work well with your particular body, how many are best for you to eat in a day, and the different ways of combining them with other foods, you will appreciate carbohydrates for what they are: a great source of energy.

WHAT ARE CARBS?

The technical definition of a carbohydrate doesn't do it a whole lot of justice: "Compounds composed of carbon, oxygen, and hydrogen arranged as monosaccharides or multiples of monosaccharides.

Most have a ration of one carbon molecule to one water molecule" (Whitney & Rolfes, 2002, p. 93). Carbohydrates are a type of nutrient that gives you energy as your body breaks it apart and uses its basic units as fuel. Carbohydrates provide 4.2 calories per gram (protein provides 4.4 and fat, 9).

Carbohydrates are classified as either simple or complex. Simple carbohydrates are broken down much more quickly than complex carbohydrates, so they are great if you need a quick source of energy (such as juice, flour, sugars). For more sustained energy, complex carbohydrates are superior because it takes our body time to break the many bonds into basic units (such as veggies and legumes). Some people's bodies break down carbs extremely quickly and find that when they eat carbs, it increases their appetite. Other people have the opposite response and feel satisfied when they eat carbs.

Knowing which category, you fall into will be very important for you to know—find out which metabolic type® you are so you know which carbs and how many are best for you.

FIBER

There are two types of fiber: soluble and insoluble. Soluble fibers dissolve in water, add bulk to stool, can decrease cholesterol and slow the absorption of glucose in the small intestines (Bland et al., 1999, p. 27). Major sources of soluble fiber are apples, oats, citrus fruits, barley and legumes. Insoluble fiber does not dissolve in water and therefore acts like a bristle brush along our intestinal wall. It adds bulk to stool and is valuable for regular bowel movements (speeds things along). Major sources of insoluble fiber are grains such as whole grain breads and cereals, wheat and corn bran, and vegetables such as cabbage, carrots, and Brussels sprouts (Whitney & Rolfes, 2002, p. 99).

TYPES OF CARBOHYDRATES

Bear with me for a moment on some technical explaining (if you really don't care, then please feel free to skip ahead to the next section). The two main categories of simple carbohydrates are monosaccharides and disaccharides. There are three types of monosaccharides and three types of disaccharides. The three types of monosaccharides are:

- Glucose--an essential energy source, also known as "blood sugar"
- Fructose--the sweetest of the sugars, found in fruits and honeys
- Galactose--combines with glucose to form lactose; milk sugar

The three types of disaccharides are:

- Maltose (glucose + glucose), produced whenever starch breaks down such as in digestion
- Sucrose (glucose + fructose), commonly known as table sugar, beet sugar or cane sugar, naturally occurring in many fruits, some vegetables and grains
- Lactose (glucose + galactose), the main carbohydrate found in milk

These simple units form the six simple carbohydrates in human nutrition. As you can see, glucose is the common thread in these carb units and is necessary for life. It is the only source of energy that the brain cells can use. Without carbohydrates, our body will convert other food sources (such as protein) into glucose. But more on this later.

As I mentioned, complex carbohydrates are similar to simple carbohydrates because they use the same basic units. The main difference is that there are many of these basic units strung together to form complex carbs or polysaccharides. Three polysaccharides that are important in nutrition are:

- Glycogen--many glucose molecules linked together and stored in the liver and muscles
- Starches--many glucose molecules linked together and stored in plants
- Fibers--non-starch polysaccharides, gives structure to plants. The main difference between starches and fibers are the digestibility. We cannot, for the most part, digest fiber.

Knowing the different mono and polysaccharides is useful when understanding nutrition because it can help you choose different foods for different situations. If you need quick energy, you know that simple carbs are better. They will raise your blood sugar quickly. If you want a more gradual rise in your energy level and more sustained energy, complex carbs are better than simple carbs.

71

Remember that your response to carbs, simple or complex, can vary tremendously from the response of another person. For example, some people do very poorly when they eat any type of carb and will crash shortly after eating them. If this describes you, another option is combining simple carbohydrates with protein or fat-rich foods. Both proteins and fats are digested more slowly and therefore will stabilize blood sugar levels, preventing spikes and crashes from occurring.

You will need to listen to your body and see which combinations make you feel the best. Some people are more sensitive than others when it comes to blood sugar balance. Listen to the signals your body gives off after eating (Do you feel jittery? Tired? Overly full? Still hungry? Balanced? Bloated?). It takes time to tune into your body, so be patient, write down if you notice feeling especially good or bad and which foods you ate (write them all down, don't just guess which food you think it was). Over time, you will notice a pattern with certain foods or food combinations. These observations are all part of learning about your unique self so that you can navigate through life making the best choices for you and not just playing a guessing game.

NUTRIENTS FOUND IN CARBS

Carbohydrates provide an array of nutrients including B Vitamins, Vitamin C, A, D, E, and K and most minerals including iron, potassium, magnesium, calcium, selenium and phosphorus. The more a food is processed, the more nutrients it loses, so aim for fresh foods as close to their original state as possible.

CARBS AND YOUR LIVER

The liver and muscles store carbohydrates as glycogen (strings of glucose). The liver stores one third of the body's total glycogen and our muscles store the other two thirds. When our blood sugar rises, the liver and muscles take the excess of whatever the cells cannot use and links the leftover glucose into chains: glycogen. When our blood sugar drops, glycogen is broken back down into glucose to be taken up by our cells. Note that our bodies do this regardless of whether we have eaten recently, which is an important survival tool. This tool also exemplifies just how important carbohydrates are to our bodies and why it is important to eat regularly and not skip meals lest you deplete your glycogen stores. The liver only holds about four hours worth of glycogen before it will start breaking down muscle tissue and converting the protein into glucose.

CARBS AND YOUR BRAIN

The brain cells can use glucose or ketones (from fat) as an energy source. The best source of glucose is from carbohydrates. If you are trying to be your healthiest, lose weight, get the most nutrition from your meal, and/or balance blood sugar, choose the best carbohydrates you can (leafy greens, veggies, fruits, and whole grains) and cut out refined carbs such as bleached flours and grains with added sweeteners. These are worlds apart in nutritional value and yet they have become synonymous. Don't make this mistake—not all carbs are created equal!

PROBLEMS WITH CARBS

Lactose Intolerance

Lactose intolerance is the most common food allergy, affecting about 10% of Americans (90-95% in African American individuals worldwide and 20-25% in Caucasian individuals) (retrieved from http://www.scienceinafrica.co.za/2002/may/milk.htm). A milk allergy is much less common. First, let me explain the difference between a "true food allergy" and a "food intolerance" (a.k.a. delayed food allergy).

We have four main pathways for fighting allergies. Different parts of our immune system respond depending on whether an allergy is immediate or delayed. A true food allergy involves an immediate immune system response every time a certain food is eaten.

Immediate-response food allergies use the Type 1 of IgE pathway. Delayed food allergies or food intolerances/sensitivities use Type 3 and 4 pathways. Delayed food allergies cause us to have a bad reaction when a certain food is eaten up to seven days later. Usually with a food intolerance, the food that causes a bad reaction needs to be eaten frequently or in large amounts before it will elicit notice-able symptoms even though damage is being done.

Some symptoms of both food allergies and intolerances are similar (nausea, diarrhea, stomach pain, headaches, fatigue) but food allergy symptoms can be a lot more serious (chest pain, shortness of breath, hives, itching skin, and anaphylactic shock).

As I was saying, a true milk allergy is less common than lactose intolerance. However, both milk allergies and lactose intolerance are even rarer if you take the method of milk processing into consideration. You have already learned the important difference between real milk (a.k.a. raw milk) and commercial milk (pasteurized, homogenized milk). Raw milk contains living beneficial bacteria and enzymes which aid in our digestion of milk. Pasteurization kills these beneficial components and therefore alters the effect the milk has on our digestive and immune system (remember that the bacteria in milk are killed by the heat in pasteurization and the dead cell bodies of the bacteria cause our body to react by releasing histamine). Many people who thought they had a milk allergy or an intolerance find that they can drink raw milk without any digestive upset!

Wheat Allergies

Wheat allergies are more common than you might think (eighth most common food allergy). You may even have a wheat allergy yourself and not know it! Although wheat allergies rarely cause life threatening symptoms such as anaphylactic shock, the symptoms are inconvenient and bothersome: digestive problems, congestion, skin irritation, and lack of energy.

Gluten Intolerance and Celiac Disease

Gluten is a protein found in grains such as wheat and barley.

Gluten contains a protein called gliadin. People who have a genetic inability to digest gliadin are called Celiacs. When a Celiac ingests gliadin, their small intestine launches an autoimmune reaction.

Usually, in order to be diagnosed with Celiac disease, a blood allergy test will be done to confirm the immune system mediators are present; however, some doctors will look at a biopsy of the small intestine.

Celiacs usually have a much more difficult time dietarily since gluten and gliadin hide in all sorts of common food additives such as food thickeners, soy sauce, hydrolyzed vegetable protein, and natural flavorings. Avoidance of problematic foods is the only way to avoid symptoms. If you suffer from gas, bloating, irregular bowel movements, or fatigue, you should get a blood test to rule out this disease.

Grain Options for Celiacs

Grains/foods that do not contain gluten are buckwheat, millet, quinoa, corn, sorghum, teff, amaranth (which contains a minute amount of gluten that is usually processed away), and all types of rice.

If you suspect you are a Celiac or have been diagnosed with Celiac disease, avoid the following grains: wheat, oats, barley, kamut, rye, spelt, semolina, bran, bulgur, couscous, and triticale.

Most health food stores carry gluten-free foods. In addition, you can find gluten-free foods at many regular grocery stores as well as online. A few online gluten-free stores are:

http://www.glutensolutions.com/
http://www.glutenfreemall.com/, and

http://www.wellnessgrocer.com/.

GLYCEMIC EFFECT OF FOOD

All foods have an effect on our blood sugar and some have more of an effect than others. The glycemic effect refers to how much a food raises our blood sugar and elicits an insulin response compared with pure glucose (Whitney & Rolfes, 2002, p. 108). If a food raises a person's blood sugar quickly and intensely, it has a high glycemic effect. The glycemic index is a list of different foods according to the degree of their glycemic effect. Ideally, if we avoid foods that cause a large surge in our blood sugar (and a resulting large surge in insulin), we will have an easier time losing weight and maintaining a healthy weight.

Problems with the Glycemic Index

There are a few flaws with the glycemic index approach. Firstly, there is some disagreement about assigned glycemic values (the test isn't always repeatable), and therefore it cannot be guaranteed that the glycemic index is accurate. Secondly, it is not scientifically agreed that the glycemic index offers any health benefits and some very healthful foods appear undesirable based solely on the index (e.g., watermelon, corn, sweet potatoes, etc.). Thirdly and most importantly, the glycemic index does not account for foods eaten together in a meal (only as single foods) and so it isn't very relevant for real-life eating situations.

TIPS FOR GLYCEMIC BALANCE

Some people are much more sensitive than others to high- glycemic and/or starchy carbohydrates and may notice a difference when they stick to low-glycemic foods. Fat and protein slow the break-down of carbohydrates and lowers the overall rise in blood sugar when eaten in the same meal. To be on the safe side, I encourage you to follow my aforementioned suggestion of eating combined foods (not carbs by themselves unless you know that your body can handle it well), and test out foods of varying glycemic levels to see which gives you lasting energy.

A SWEET DEBATE: SUGAR VERSUS STEVIA

Sugar and artificial sweeteners have become a real health problem for people. They are used in so many items besides sweets that it is actually harder to find breads, cereals, drinks and snack foods that don't have added sweeteners. I have dedicated a lot of time and research to sugar alternatives. In a recent study, artificial sweeteners were found to hinder weight loss by disrupting one's ability to regulate caloric intake (Swithers & Davidson, 2008).

Rather than focusing on all artificial sweeteners and sugar alternatives, I would instead like to educate you on my favorite sugar alternative: stevia. Many people have never heard of it or haven't used it and instead use artificial sweeteners, which are questionable at best, in terms of their effect on our health. Stevia is a leafy green plant (Asteraceae family, genus Stevia, species rebaudiana) that was identified and classified by Dr. Moises Santiago Bertoni in the late 1800s, but its use by the Guarani Indians in South America dates back centuries (Kirkland, J. and T., 2002).

HEALTH BENEFITS OF STEVIA

Stevia is a natural sweetener that does not raise your blood sugar and it adds no calories to the diet. It is 250-300 times sweeter than table sugar and stable to 392 degrees Fahrenheit. Unlike sugar, stevia has many health benefits including:

- Preventing cavities and gum disease by inhibiting the growth of some bacteria and infectious organisms
- Improving digestion
- Balancing blood glucose levels
- Balancing blood pressure
- Improving skin conditions such as acne, seborrhea, dermatitis, and eczema
- Aiding in weight loss

It is no surprise that stevia is gaining in popularity worldwide.

Aside from being a great sweetener, it is sold in some South American countries as an aid to people with diabetes and hypoglycemia (May, 2007).

Weight Loss Management with Stevia

Stevia is also an exceptional aid in weight loss management because it contains no calories and reduces the craving for sweets. Stevio-sides, the principle sugar molecule component of stevia, pass un-changed through our digestive tract and are not absorbed into the blood, therefore producing no calories. Some preliminary research indicates that stevia may actually "reset" the hunger mechanism in people who have trouble between the part of their brain which controls hunger--the hypothalamus--and their stomach. By resetting this communication pathway, the body is able to reduce feelings of hunger more quickly (retrieved from www.happystomach.com).

Using Stevia

For sweetening drinks and non-baked foods, stevia is easy to use and comes in several forms (packets, liquid, and bulk powder).

Remember that with stevia, a little goes a long way. Taste as you go. For a large mug of hot tea, I usually use only ¼-½ teaspoon. If you frequently go to coffee shops and drink coffee or tea, I recommend buying liquid stevia. It has a dropper in the lid to make it convenient to add to drinks (so don't have to worry about blending as much).

You still get the sweet taste without all the calories and negative health effects of sugar.

The main drawback of stevia is that it doesn't cook the same as sugar: it cannot caramelize, add volume or texture, and if you use too much, whatever you are making will taste bitter rather than sweet. In summary, you have to practice cooking with it, but the health benefits are well worth it. There are many online cookbooks and published books for details on cooking with stevia. A fantastic book is Sugar-Free Cooking with Stevia by James and Tanya Kirkland. It contains plenty of yummy recipes and hints for successfully replacing sugar/sweeteners with stevia.

Stevia Safety

Stevia is a safe sugar alternative. It has a long track record of safety—1500 years, in fact. Following extensive research, Dr. Daniel Mowrey reported:

More elaborate safety tests were performed by the Japanese during their evaluation of stevia as a possible sweetening agent. Few substances have ever yielded such consistently negative results in toxicity trials as have stevia. Almost every toxicity test imaginable has been performed on stevia extract [concentrate] or stevioside at one time or another. The results are always negative. No abnormalities in weight change, food intake, cell or membrane characteristics, enzyme and substrate utilization, or chromosome characteristics. No cancer, no birth defects, no acute and no chronic untoward effects. Nothing. (retrieved from http://www.healthynet.com)

To read some of the many various safety studies and comments by doctors, herbalists, and scientists, visit www.stevia.net/safety.

Here you can also read about how the rumors of stevia's "contraceptive effects" got started and why they are invalid. This rumor has not once been shown in any lab study. Search for yourself! Instead you will find numerous studies of the benefits of stevia and join the many hopefuls that stevia will soon be used on a commercial scale as a sugar alternative...it's starting at least.

TRUVIA™

For baking, you can also try Truvia™: a product that uses Rebiana and erythritol. Rebiana is the "best tasting part of the stevia plant" and erythritol is a sugar alcohol. Truvia™ is granulated and comes in packets. One packet contains the same sweetness as two teaspoons of sugar and just like stevia, it is a zero calorie sweetener. It is easy to cook and bake with, tastes great and is quickly gaining in popularity and therefore widely available. Go to www.truvia.com for recipes.

LAKANTO, ERYTHRITOL, & MONK FRUIT

Lakanto is the closest natural sweetener to sugar in terms of its taste and its usability. The two natural ingredients in Lakanto are non-GMO erythritol and the super sweet extract of the luo han guo fruit (aka monk fruit, used in China for centuries). This fruit's extract is 300 times sweeter than table sugar!

Erythritol is better than other sugar alcohols because it is fermented. The erythritol in Lakanto is made by fermenting the sugar in non-GMO corn. Similar to xylitol, people can have diarrhea, gas and bloating with foods sweetened with sugar alcohols, but this tends not to be a problem with Lakanto. This may be because Lakanto is processed differently (fermented versus hydrogenated).

Health Benefits of Lakanto

- Zero calories
- Zero additives
- No influence on your blood sugar and insulin (safe for diabetics)
- A one-to-one ratio with sugar so it's easy to measure and use in baking

It appears that if you aren't cooking and baking with it, monk fruit works well as a sweetener and tends to be less processed than Lakanto. There are no reported negative effects~in fact, there are some health benefits associated with monk fruit such as inhibiting tumor growth, antioxidant, anti-inflammatory, and blood pressure regulation (all similar to stevia, except the aftertaste). As far as versatility with recipes, Lakanto has benefits over monk fruit.

If you are struggling with sugar addiction, Lakanto or monk fruit looks promising as a replacement. As with any sweetener, moderation is recommended and if you do try it and your body language tells you that it doesn't agree with you, please listen!

D-TAGATOSE

A fairly new sweetener that has promise, D-tagatose is derived from milk sugar. Because it is incompletely digested, it has about 75% fewer calories than sugar.

Blood Sugar Effect

Because tagatose is incompletely absorbed, it only slightly raises blood sugar and insulin levels. It has been confirmed in several clinical studies to be a low glycemic sweetener and have a low glycemic effect.

One study even showed no increase in glucose or insulin in people with either Type II diabetes or people with normal blood sugar regulation. Tagatose appears to be a great sweetening alternative for people interested in keeping blood sugar levels steady (which is most of us!).

Prebiotic Effect

Clinical research has shown that tagatose acts as a prebiotic.

When test subjects consumed tagatose, their "good" bacteria in the large intestine and colon increased. These strains of bacteria are essential to maintaining a healthy digestive system.

Lower in Calories Than Sugar

Because tagatose is incompletely digested, it only 1.5 calories per gram, whereas sugar has 4 calories per gram. For food labeling purposes in the US, the low caloric value allows tagatose to say it is both "zero calorie" and, as long as the serving stays .5 grams or less, the label can also claim that it is "sugar-free."

Does Not Promote Tooth Decay

Like Stevia, tagatose does not promote dental caries as regular sugar does. Studies show that after eating tagatose, the processes that promote tooth decay do not occur.

Recommended Fiber Intake

The standard fiber recommendation is between 25-30 grams per day. This recommendation falls short on many counts. The world-wide average fiber intake is between 50-75 grams and studies in countries where fiber intake is even higher (75-100 grams) suggest that higher fiber levels are healthy for us. Unfortunately, fiber intake in the United States is below 10 grams a day (Bland, et al., 1999, p. 27).

Fiber is extremely important to our digestive and cardiovascular health by regulating bowel movements and acting as a vehicle for carrying extra cholesterol out of the body. It plays a key role in blood sugar regulation and cancer protection (Bland, et al., 1999) by its ability to slow down gastric emptying and improve overall health.

As with every other nutrient, the exact amount of fiber we should ingest each day depends on our biochemistry. Eating some raw veggies or greens such as spinach or lettuce daily is a good idea for most people (see the next section for potential negative side effects), but regular bowel movements and healthy hearts are certainly possible on a diet high in protein and fat. Weston Price's anthropological efforts uncovered civilizations such as the Inuits who thrive on mostly animal fat and protein and almost no carbohydrates. The Masai tribe in Africa depend heavily on cow's blood, milk and meat. In his 1841 Polynesian expedition, Captain Charles Wilkes discovered that the Tokelau natives lived on a mostly fish and coconut diet (Taubes, 2007). Clearly, fiber in and of itself is not what constitutes a healthy diet. Rather, the right mixture of proteins, fats, and carbs are more important when it comes to the big "health" picture.

THE BEST CARBS

Unless you have a particular digestive condition or an allergy to any food from the carbohydrate family, the best carbohydrates are complex carbohydrates. Depending on your unique body, you may do better with cooked veggies or fruit versus raw, and certain food combinations (e.g., eating meat with grains as opposed to fruit), etc.

When it comes down to it, listen to your body. If you feel fatigued, bloated, gassy, or queasy after eating certain foods or food combinations, you should talk to a nutritionist or other appropriate health professional to investigate a food intolerance or possible digestive issue.

Also, depending on your unique body chemistry, you may feel better with more carbohydrates than other people or far less carbs than other people. This is a situation best handled by paying attention to how you feel one to two hours after eating. Finding out your metabolic type® can be a tremendous help in determining the right food choices and amounts for you. Knowing your metabolic type® will take a lot of the guesswork out of food selection and food combining.

Having said all that, here are some of the top carbohydrates you should experiment with incorporating into your diet to improve your health:

- Vegetables such as broccoli, cauliflower, cabbage, Brussels sprouts, kohlrabi, carrots (full-grown carrots with the skins on them have B12 if you are careful not to scrub them too much when washing), mushrooms, jicama, potatoes (red and purple have less starch), onions, leeks, squash, zucchini, artichokes, and green beans.

- Leafy greens such as spinach, romaine, kale, chard, beet greens, turnip greens, collard greens, endive.

- Fruits such as apples, coconut, grapefruit, kiwi, watermelon, figs, lemons, limes, oranges, raspberries, blueberries, strawberries, cranberries, pomegranate, pears, cherries, peaches, apricots, nectarines, goji berries, and grapes.

- Legumes such as beans, peas, and lentils.

- Gluten-free grains and pseudo-grains such as brown, black, or wild rice, oats, quinoa, buckwheat, amaranth, teff, millet, and sorghum.

Choosing Quality Carbs

1. I will observe which carbohydrates I eat this week and write down how I feel after eating them (e.g., broccoli, satisfied, good energy).

2. I choose to eat complex carbohydrates. I will eat one veggie that I don't normally eat and write down if I react positively or negatively to it (e.g., zucchini, positive reaction).

3. I will use a healthy alternative sweetener as a substitute for sugar this week, eat at least three salads this week, and write down two or more top carbs I think I digest well.

Chapter 6

Fats

F'ats are essential nutrients that provide our bodies with the means to build healthy cells, insulate and protect vital organs, manufacture hormones, provide energy, help regulate blood pressure and inflammation, contribute to healthy skin and eyes, and aid in proper brain development. Without the right fats in our diet, we would basically cease to exist.

Because fats are high in calories (nine calories per gram--more than twice the calories per gram in either carbohydrates or proteins), we have come to fear fat and exclude it from our diets. What I hope to teach you in this chapter is how vital good fats are for your health and how by eating the right fats in the right amounts, you will actually lose weight, have more energy, and feel satisfied rather than deprived, after eating. Before we get into specific fats that you should have in your diet, let's first take a look at the structure of a fatty acid. (Feel free to skip ahead if this doesn't interest you.)

FATTY ACIDS

When you talk about dietary fats, you are really talking about fatty acids (an organic compound of a carbon chain with hydrogens at one end--the fatty chain--and an acid group at the other end). The fatty chain end of the fatty acid is fat-soluble and water-insoluble, but the acid end is the opposite: fat-insoluble and water-soluble (Erasmus, 1993). Fatty acids, or fats, can vary in ways that drastically change their effect on our bodies. Length, degree of unsaturation, and location of double bonds (two carbon atoms) all determine whether or not a fat is healthy for us.

Fatty Acid Length

Fatty acids can be long or short. The most common short fatty acid length is between four carbons long--butyric acid, or butter-- and the longest is twenty-four carbons long--fish oil and brain tissue (Erasmus, 1993, p. 15). Short-chain and medium-chain saturated fatty acids like coconut and palm kernel oil are very easy to digest and are a preferred fat for people with digestive problems or liver ailments.

Longer-chain saturated fats (beef, pork) are solid at room temperature and take longer to digest. Long-chain saturated fatty acids have many functions in the body. They are used as building blocks to build strong cell walls, protect our liver from alcohol and other toxins, are needed for proper use of essential fatty acids and much more. Our bodies prefer to use the softer short- and medium- chain fats for energy and not storage (e.g., on your rear end!).

$$\begin{array}{ccccccccc} H & H & H & H & H & & H & H & H & H \\ | & | & | & | & | & & | & | & | & | \\ H-C-C-C-C-C & = & C-C-C-C-COOH \\ | & | & | & | & & & | & | & | \\ H & H & H & H & & & H & H & H \end{array}$$

Monounsaturated

As the example shows, the degree of saturation is an important determinant in the function of a fat. The more saturated a fatty acid, the more stable it is: the more unsaturated it is, the more chemically active it is. Saturated fatty acids have all of their carbon atoms bonded with hydrogen atoms and all of these bonds are single bonds. A monounsaturated fatty acid has all of its carbons bonded with hydrogens except one (which is missing two hydrogens) and one of its carbons has a double bond. Polyunsaturated fatty acids have two or more double bonds.

$$H-C-C = C-C-C = C-C-C-C-COOH$$

Polyunsaturated

Polyunsaturated fats are named according to their omega; the location of their first double bond in relation to the fatty end of the fatty acid (i.e., methyl end). For instance, an omega-3 fatty acid is a fatty acid with its first double bond three carbons away from the methyl end. Likewise, an omega-6 fatty acid has its first double bond six carbons away from the methyl end.

OMEGA-3'S VERSUS OMEGA-6'S

Both Omega-3 and Omega-6 oils' fatty acids are essential fatty acids, or EFAs for short. Both are absolutely required for health and we must get them from our diet since our bodies are unable to make them. Ideally, you want about a tablespoon of Omega-6 fats per day and 1-2 teaspoons of Omega-3 fats. It is common that we get too much Omega-6 and not enough Omega-3 fats in our diets. We should aim for a four to one ratio of Omega-6 to Omega-3 oils in our diet.

Omega-3 fats (aka alpha-linolenic acid or LNA) are amongst the healthiest dietary fats. (Just as we refine wheat to make flour to use in breads, cereals and crackers, LNA can be metabolized into stearidonic acid (SDA), eicosapentaenoic acid (EPA), and/or docosahexaenoic acid (DHA).) They are found in flax, hemp seed, walnut, soybean, dark leafy greens, black currant seed, salmon, trout, mackerel, sardines, and

Chinese water snake oil (Erasmus, 1993, p.22). Because Omega-3s are so chemically active, they are used in many functions throughout the body including faster recovery from fatigue, prostaglandin (cellular mechanics) production, increasing growth and metabolic rate, proper cell division, keeping membranes fluid, brain development, proper immune function, reducing inflammation.

An important side note that you won't read about in most health books is how Omega-3 fats are very delicate and are easily damaged by oxygen. Without sufficient antioxidants such as vitamin C and E, these Omega-3 fats become free radicals and actually increase aging and damage to your cells.

Omega-6 fats (aka linoleic acid or LA) are abundant in safflower, corn, sunflower, borage, evening primrose, and sesame oils. (LA can be metabolized into gamma-linolenic acid (GLA), dihomogamma linolenic acid (DGLA), and arachidonic acid (AA).) Omega-6 fats, like Omega-3s, aid in metabolism, energy conversion, and growth.

Blood Stickiness

One of the most important differences between Omega-3s and Omega 6s is their effect on our blood: Omega-3 fats keep our blood fluid and less sticky whereas Omega-6s help our blood to clot by increasing its stickiness. Both are important functions, but you can see how necessary it is to keep a proper ratio of the two so that our blood maintains proper stickiness (Aukerman, 2007).

Inflammation Regulation

Another important difference between Omega-3 and Omega-6 fats is their effect on inflammation. The main Omega-3 fats category, Alpha-linolenic Acid (LNA), have an anti-inflammatory effect on the body because they are used to make Series 1 and 3 prostaglandins (little hormone-like chemicals that act like universal body mechanics). Omega-6 fats can have both an anti-inflammatory effect and an inflammatory effect since one of their pathways (AA) is used to make Series 2 prostaglandins: Series 2 prostaglandins can lead to increased inflammation, water retention, and increased blood pressure (Erasmus, 1993).

SATURATED FATS

For years I have heard about how bad saturated fats are for humans, how we don't need saturated fats, and how they contribute to heart disease and cancer. However, there is actually a substantial amount of evidence to the contrary. Did you know that saturated fats have been in our diets for seven million years!

Certain metabolic types® THRIVE on saturated fats. Studies of Eskimos, North American Indians, and other tribes suggest that they ingested as much as 80% of their daily calories from fat, and mostly from saturated animal fat (Fallon & Enig, 2007, www.westonaprice. org).

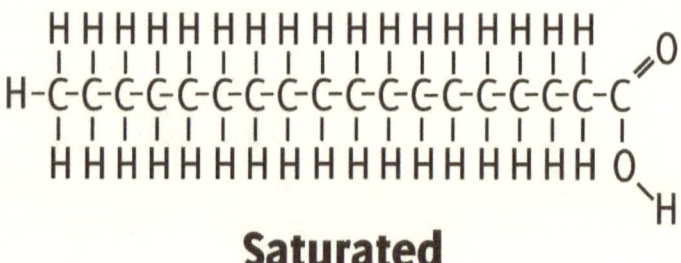

Saturated

Coconut oil, organic ghee and butter, as well as fats from healthy animals are very important for optimal health. In 1998, the World Health Organization collected data on a large international scale, looking at heart disease deaths and saturated fat consumption--and guess what they found, much to their chagrin? The seven countries with the least saturated fat intake had more deaths from heart disease than every single one of the seven countries with the highest saturated fat intake! (Kendrick, 2008).

We have been told that saturated fats are to blame for heart disease, but the facts do not support this theory. The opposite is true. Looking at data between 1910-1970 clearly shows that we had less heart disease when we ate more animal fat. The 20% decline in butter consumption and the large increase in vegetable oil consumption has led to heart disease being the leading cause of death in Americans today. Remember that we have been eating saturated animal fats for millions of years. They cannot be blamed for modern diseases.

Clearly the role of saturated fats in our diet is being misunderstood. We need to get back to eating these beneficial fats. As with all fats, the quality makes a huge difference in how the fat will affect your health. See later in this chapter for some suggestions.

CHOLESTEROL MYTH

Cholesterol is a necessary substance made by our liver to build and repair cell walls. Cholesterol has gotten a bad wrap for a long time yet we know now it does NOT cause heart disease.

So why has cholesterol been blamed for heart disease all these years? It's a very long story! In a nutshell, it is analogous to a paramedic showing up at the scene of an accident to help and then being blamed later for causing the accident. Just because cholesterol is present in blocked arteries does not mean it is to blame for the underlying issue.

Recently, more and more peer reviewed medical journals published reports stating that they've been wrong about both saturated fat AND cholesterol being the cause of heart disease. Both are necessary in the diet and they aren't "bad" for you. What is bad for you is too much sugar and refined carbohydrates (bread, cereal, crackers, chips, etc.). When we eat too many of these foods, insulin and inflammation go up increasing your body's likelihood of becoming insulin-resistant (as with Type-2 diabetes), storing more body fat and damaging arteries along the way. Cholesterol comes to the rescue and attempts to repair the damage, but if it can't or if the cause of inflammation continues (poor diet, too much sugar and carbs), heart disease may develop.

As you can see, high cholesterol is merely a symptom of an underlying imbalance and recovery from fatigue; however, there are some key differences between the essential fatty acids.

How Much Fat Do We Need?

Some people thrive on a high fat diet while others do not. There is no perfect amount of fat for everyone. Government dietary guidelines are that we need about 20-35% of our daily calories from fat.

*In instances of arterial blockage and other degenerative disease, some diets recommend as little as 10% of total calories to come from fat. Once regression of the disease is noticed, a higher fat intake ensues. This approach may work for some people, but makes other people sicker (former President Eisenhower is a perfect example).

Continuing a very low fat intake is not recommended and can be dangerous.

Aim for the best fats you can—the less refined, the better. Find out how much fat is ideal for you by paying close attention to how you feel after eating. After eating meals that match your nutrient ratio properly, you should feel satisfied, energetic, and mentally clear.

Again, identifying your metabolic type® can be a tremendous help and take a lot of the guesswork out of eating and food combining for you.

Best Dietary Fats

Having stated the disclaimer that there are certain healthy fats and oils that won't necessarily match your unique biochemistry, below are some great recommendations to work with. Choose fats and oils from this list and over time, observe which ones make you feel the best:

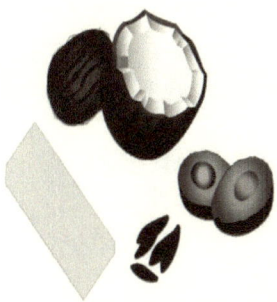

- Get yourself some flax oil in a dark container (light damages essential fatty acids, as does heat and oxygen) and keep it in the refrigerator. Take one teaspoon a day either on salad, fruit, yogurt, etc., or by itself.

- Eat fish 2-3 times per week. If you take a fish oil supplement, take a good quality krill oil.

- Excellent brands for essential fatty acids are Nordic Naturals, Rosita, Udo's Oils, Pharmax Finest, and Budwig's Flax Oil/Coconut Fat Spread.

- Regularly buy a variety of seeds and nuts. The longer you keep them, the more their fats break down. If you enjoy the taste, opt for raw nuts and seeds as the heat used to roast them speeds up the breakdown and health benefits of their fats. Aim for a small handful a day (some metabolic types® require more).

WHAT HAPPENS WHEN YOU DON'T GET ENOUGH FAT?

Because fats are so critical for cellular formation and stability, growth, metabolism, and more, our body doesn't take too kindly when we deprive ourselves of sufficient healthy fats. Did you know that your liver can make fat? It can, and does, make saturated fat if quality fats are not consumed in your diet (or if you eat too many refined, sugary carbohydrates). Many other liver problems arise without proper fat intake. In as little as four weeks of a fat-free diet, symptoms of essential fatty acid deficiency will begin (see chart), metabolism slows down, and the body gains weight more easily (Cabot, 1996).

Signs of Fatty Acid Deficiency

LA (Omega 6)	ALA (Omega 3)
Loss of hair	High blood pressure
Sticky platelets	High triglycerides
Behavioral disturbances	Poor motor coordination
Liver or kidney degeneration	Learning impairment
Excessive sweating with thirst	Tingling arms and legs
Eczema-like skin eruptions	Dry skin or edema
Poor wound healing	Immune dysfunction
Susceptibility to infections	Behavioral changes
Sterility (males)/miscarriage	Growth retardation
Heart/Circulatory problems	Mental deterioration

BUYING THE BEST OIL

Many of the oils sold in grocery stores are unhealthy, processed and rancid. They barely even resemble the life-giving fats that they started out as. Bleaching, deodorizing, and degumming are only a few of the steps in the process of oil refinement that damage the oils and deplete their nutrients. Here are some steps that you can take to ensure that you are getting a good quality oil:

- Always buy oil in opaque containers like colored glass or metal. Clear glass lets light in, which damages the oil. The longer it sits on the shelf in the grocery store exposed to light, the less healthful it will be. The darker the glass, the less light gets in.

- Buy oils that say unrefined, virgin, or extra-virgin on the bottle or label.

- Oils that have been mechanically pressed (expeller pressed) are better than oils that have been chemically pressed (no solvent residue). The term cold-pressed does not mean that an oil is healthy: it just means that no additional heat (aside from the heat created by the friction of pressing the seed or nut) was used during the oil extraction process.

Trans Fats

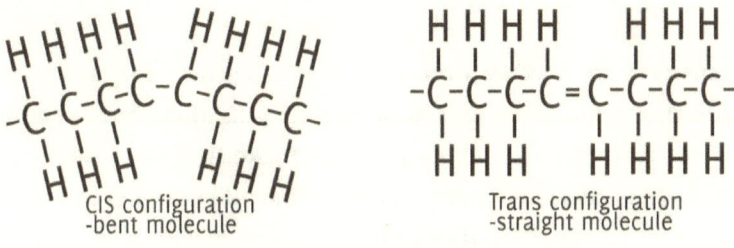

CIS configuration
-bent molecule

Trans configuration
-straight molecule

CIS Fat vs. Trans Fat

The worst fats are trans fats: fats that have been chemically modified (to add hydrogen) so that their shape changes and the fatty acid is twisted. Normal fats are arranged in a cis-configuration, not a trans-configuration: the hydrogens that attach to the carbons of the double bond in a fatty acid are on the same side, creating a bend.

Trans fats have one hydrogen on one side and the other hydrogen on the opposite side. This small change in shape results in a functionally very different fat that can wreak havoc on our body. When we try to use trans fats the way we would use healthy fats in our bodies, it is similar to using cake frosting instead of grout between tiles. Trans fats fill the physical space of cis fats, but they cannot perform the functions of cis fats. Trans fats are cis fat impersonators.

95

TRANS FATS AND CHOLESTEROL

Research has shown that trans fats can increase our blood cholesterol levels by up to 15%, our blood fat or triglycerides by up to 47%, increase the size of plaque in our arteries, increase LDL (typically referred to as bad cholesterol) AND decrease our HDL (typically referred to as good cholesterol), increase Lp(a) (worst cholesterol), increase our incidence of cancer, decrease insulin response, interfere with essential fatty acid metabolism, and more (Erasmus, 1993).

Seriously, trans fats have no business being in your body. The damages they are known to cause may be just the tip of the iceberg.

Avoiding Trans Fats

Trans fats are used in processed foods because they have a longer shelf life (trans fats are more saturated, making them more stable) and creamy texture (adding hydrogens to make it more saturated and firmer). Some trans fats occur naturally in small amounts in meat, milk, and butter; but most of them are found in margarines, shortenings, processed foods, and partially or fully hydrogenated vegetable oils.

To avoid most trans fats, read labels before buying and avoid products that contain partially hydrogenated and hydrogenated oils in the ingredients. You cannot just look at the "Nutrition Facts" section on the food label because if there are .5 grams or less trans fats per serving, the label will say zero trans fats. This may not seem like much, but considering the damage trans fats can do to our health, any amount is bad for us. Moreover, if you eat several servings or several foods that have .5 grams of trans fats, they add up quickly over the day, week, month, etc.

OTHER FATS TO AVOID

Damaged fats are best avoided. Fats get damaged in a variety of ways:

- Light
- Oxygen
- Heat

All of these produce free radicals--electrons that aren't paired and will steal electrons from other pairs of molecules. Free radicals are thought to be a main cause of aging and degenerative disease. They damage our cells by bumping into them and trying to steal electrons. When they bump into our cells, chain reactions can occur if we don't have adequate antioxidants to stop all the molecules from losing electrons. Antioxidants such as Vitamin C, E, bioflavanoids and carotene are very important for protecting our bodies against free radical damage (Erasmus, 1993).

When oils are exposed to light, oxygen, and heat, free radicals are produced. If we ingest these oils, we are increasing the free radicals in our bodies and inviting the opportunity for them to damage our cells That is why it is so important to take in quality oils--those that have been handled carefully to reduce free radical production--and to treat the oils with caution so they don't oxidize and become a danger to us.

BEST Cooking Oils

Some trans fats are also created through high-heat cooking or frying. It is recommended to cook at lower temperatures whenever possible. The oils that are damaged less by frying are those that are more saturated or those that are more refined.

Use the following guide to ensure you are using the right oil for your cooking needs.

COOKING OIL GUIDE

No Heat (up to 120 degrees F/49 C):

- Flax Seed
- Hemp Seed
- Borage
- Primrose

Low Heat (up to 212 F/100 C) (when baking at 350 degrees, the moisture keeps the inside temperature under 212 degrees):

- Sunflower (preferably high oleic)
- Safflower (preferably high oleic)

Medium Heat (325 F/163 C) Light sautéing:

- Butter
- Olive
- Hazelnut
- Sesame
- Peanut

High Heat (375 F/190 C) frying/browning:

- Coconut
- Ghee (clarified butter)
- Lard
- Palm oil

IMPORTANT COOKING TIP

Bear in mind that the hotter and longer oils are exposed to heat, the less beneficial they are to you. Experiment with other cooking styles like wet-frying (add water to the oil so that the temperature stays lower, around 212 degrees), boiling, steaming, or lower-heat sautéing. When frying, always put oil into the pan first and heat up gradually.

CHOOSING QUALITY FATS

1. I will throw away any margarine or trans fat product that I have and I will buy and try a quality saturated cooking fat (coconut oil, ghee, or lard).

2. I will cook with quality oils and I will add an Omega-3 fatty acid source into my daily diet such as fish, flax seeds or flax oil, walnuts and/or a krill oil supplement.

3. I will look at any processed food that I buy this week to see if it has trans fats—if it does, I will choose a trans-fat-free alternative. I will also add an Omega-3 fatty acid source into my daily diet.

Chapter 7

Proteins

When you hear the word protein, what foods come to mind? A big juicy steak? Yeah, that's what I thought! While there is nothing wrong with a big steak (for the right metabolic type®), I'd like to educate you on many protein sources so that you will have variety and can choose the sources that make you feel your best. But first, let's start at square one with what protein is.

WHAT IS PROTEIN?

Protein is a macronutrient, as are carbs and fats, whose building blocks are chains of amino acids. These basic units of protein are used for hundreds of functions throughout the body. We use amino acids to rebuild skin, hair, nails, cells, muscles; regulate fluid balance and acid-base balance in the body; serve as enzymes, antibodies and carriers for iron, fats, and other nutrients; and to convert to glucose to be used as energy if needed. Protein, because it supplies us with vital amino acids, is a key nutrient for health and we need a fresh supply of it daily since we do not store it like we store fat and carbohydrates.

RECOMMENDED PROTEIN INTAKE

Proper protein recommendation is an incredibly controversial topic. Mainstream recommendations for protein intake are based on the concept of "nitrogen balance." The concept of nitrogen balance goes something like this: Protein contains nitrogen, and as proteins are broken down in the body, nitrogen is excreted. Consequently, for the body to continue to make proteins, nitrogen must be continually replaced through the diet (as protein). An ideal nitrogen balance for most adults is an even nitrogen balance. This means that the amount of dietary nitrogen is equivalent to the amount of excreted nitrogen. For children, pregnant and lactating women, a positive nitrogen balance is required to support the increased growth and development. This means that more nitrogen (protein) needs to be taken in as food than the amount of nitrogen that is eliminated.

PROTEIN RDAS

Recommended Dietary Allowances (RDAs) are a popular way of standardizing nutrient suggestions. This sort of cookie-cutter approach is not going to apply to most of us. In real life and outside of the text books, we have all known people who seemed to thrive on a higher protein diet. Maybe you're one of them. Not everyone fits into the nice mold of "you need this many grams of protein per day."

CARNIVORES VERSUS CARBIVORES

For years I followed conventional recommendations for protein. I experimented with vegetable protein sources instead of animal sources. While that may work for some people, I can answer without a shadow of a doubt that my body is healthiest with relatively large amounts of protein. I discovered this after learning what my metabolic type® was and after a great deal of experimenting. I ended up shifting my diet dramatically. Instead of relying on carbs, I found that I had much better, sustained energy when I ate animal protein. In turn, I have advised countless clients to learn how much and which types of proteins were best for them. It is important to understand that listening to your body is some of the best research you can do.

METABOLIC TYPING® AND PROTEIN NEEDS

The human body needs protein every day to repair hair, skin, and tissues. We require more protein if we have to repair an injury, a protein absorption dysfunction, exercising for long periods of time, and if we are pregnant. The exact amount of extra protein each of us needs depends on our biochemistry. There are certain metabolic types®, however, that just thrive on protein. And not just any protein, but the fleshy animal kind.

MISSION OF PERSONAL OBSERVATION:

Do You Accept This Challenge?

First, I would highly recommend taking a metabolic typing® questionnaire. There are so many different areas that will be tested and overall you will get a much clearer, more comprehensive picture of your body and how it works. But whether you do the test or not, you will need to experiment with food to clue yourself in on which foods make you feel the best—more energy, less cravings, mental clarity, etc. This experimenting goes far beyond your enjoyment of different food types—we're not trying to figure out which foods taste the best to you. I challenge you to find out which foods leave you feeling full/satisfied, energetic, able to concentrate, emotionally balanced and without cravings, minutes after you've just finished eating.

PROTEIN AND BODYBUILDING

Many bodybuilders will argue that to put on more muscle, you need to eat a lot more protein. This simply isn't true for everyone. It is possible to over-consume protein. As few as 10-15 more grams per day will be sufficient overconsumption for many people. The most muscle the human body can build in a week is one pound— this is the upper limit of our muscle fibers' capacity to convert protein into muscle (Bailey, 1994). If you keep eating protein attempting to build more muscle than that, unless your unique biochemistry happens to assimilate protein extremely well, the added calories will be converted to fat. This will show up as extra weight on the scale. So, you might think that you have foiled your own physiology, but all you have succeeded in doing is increasing your fat stores and taxed your kidneys with extra protein.

QUALITY NOT QUANTITY

If you need more convincing, take a look at the amount of protein newborns get in their diets and the growth spurts they are able to achieve—breast milk contains wonderful quality protein, but the newborn is still only getting about 1% of its total calories per day from protein, and yet can double its birth weight in six months! (Holford, 1999). Quality of protein is more important than quantity when it comes to building muscle. The liver breaks up amino acids and assembles them in the desired pattern to make the proteins that it needs to carry out many bodily functions. As with fats and carbs, every person has certain protein foods on which their body thrives.

Let your personal discoveries do the talking. If you notice that you do better with more protein in your diet, adjust accordingly.

SOURCES OF PROTEIN

FOOD, SERVING, CALORIES. PROTEIN GRAMS]

Tamari (Soy Sauce) [1 tbs, 11 cals, 1-2g]

Romaine Lettuce [2 cup, 16, 2]

Spirulina – dried [1 tbs, 20, 4]

Mustard greens, boiled [1 cup, 21, 3]

Cauliflower, boiled [1 cup, 28, 2]

Crimini mushrooms, raw [5 oz, 31, 3.5]

Cabbage, common shredded, boiled [1 cup, 4, 2]

Swiss chard, boiled [1 cup, 35, 3]

Kale, boiled [1 cup, 36, 2-3]

Summer squash, cooked [1 cup, 36, 1.6]

Tomato, ripe [Medium, 38, 1-2]

Spinach, boiled [1 cup, 41, 5]

Garlic [1 oz, 42, 2]

Asparagus [5 spears, 43.2, 2]

Broccoli, steamed [1 cup, 43.7, 4-5]

Green beans, boiled [1 cup, 44, 2-3]

Cabbage, red, shredded; boiled [1 cup, 44, 2]

Turnip greens, cooked [1 cup, 48, 5.5]

Collard greens, boiled [1 cup, 49, 4]

Brussel's sprouts, boiled [1 cup, 56, 4]

Eggs, whole, boiled [1 each, 68, 6]

Miso [1 oz, 71, 4]

Mozzarella cheese, part skim, shredded [4 oz, 72, 6-7]

Tofu, raw [4 oz, 86, 9]

Shitake mushrooms, raw [8 oz, 87, 5]

Shrimp, steamed; boiled [4 oz, 112 cals, 24g]

Cod, baked; broiled [4 oz, 119, 26]

Cow's milk; 2 % [1 cup, 121, 8]

Green peas, boiled [1 cup, 134, 8-9]

Snapper, baked/broiled [4 oz, 145, 30]

Scallops, baked/broiled [4 oz, 152, 23]

Yogurt, low-fat, plain [1 cup, 155, 13]

Tuna, yellow fin, baked/broiled [4 oz, 157, 34]

Halibut, baked/broiled [4 oz,159, 30]

Potato (baked with skin) [Medium, 161,4]

Oats, whole grain, cooked [1 cup, 166, 6]

Goat's milk [1 cup, 168, 8-9]

Venison [4 oz, 179, 34]

Peanut Butter [2 tbs, 180, 7-9]

Calf's liver, braised [4 oz, 187, 24.5]

Pumpkin seeds, raw [¼ cup, 187, 8.5]

Almond butter [2 tbs, 190, 5-8]

Peanuts, raw [1/ cup, 207, 9]

Turkey breast, roasted [4 oz, 214, 32.5]

Lima beans, cooked [1 cup, 216, 14-15]

Rice, brown, cooked [1 cup, 216, 5]

Chicken breast, roasted [4 oz, 223, 34]

Tempeh, cooked [4 oz, 223, 21]

Kidney beans, cooked [1 cup, 225, 15]

Black beans, cooked [1 cup, 227, 15]

Lamb loin, roasted [4 oz, 229, 30]

Lentils, cooked [1 cup, 230, 17-18]

Split peas, cooked [1 cup, 231, 16]

Pinto beans, cooked [1 cup, 234, 14]

Beef tenderloin, lean, broiled [4 oz, 1 cup, 240, 32]

Spelt grains, cooked [1 cup, 246, 10-11]

Quinoa, cooked [1 cup, 254, 9]

Navy beans, cooked [1 cup, 258, 16]

Salmon, Chinook, baked/broiled [4 oz, 262, 29]

Garbanzo beans (chick peas), cooked [1 cup, 269, 14-15]

Soybeans, cooked [1 cup, 298, 29]

*USDA Nutrient Database

Most foods, except fruit, have protein. If you are eating a whole foods diet (i.e., not a lot of processed, packaged foods) then you are getting plenty of protein to survive—but you may not be getting enough to thrive. As mentioned previously, some people need quite a bit more protein in their diet to feel their best and be their healthiest.

Animal protein is more concentrated gram for gram, whereas calorie for calorie, non-meat sources contain more protein. The list shows you how much protein is in both animal and vegetable foods sorted by calories. Calories and grams are rounded to the nearest decimal point.

This list is good news if you are the type of person who doesn't do well when you eat a lot of animal protein because you can see that there are plenty of protein-dense options. If you feel better after eating animal protein, this list shows you a variety of options as well. It is important to recognize that protein is present in many different foods and it may be good to expand your repertoire of protein foods, especially when high quality animal proteins sources are not available to you.

Whether you are trying to eat less meat or not (or fewer calories or not), the truth of the matter is that some people do better when they consume higher amounts of animal protein sources compared to non-meat protein sources regardless of the caloric difference. This preference is not merely one of taste. It is much more in-depth than that. Every single food you ingest effects your biochemistry and your pH balance.

pH Balance and Meat

A well-researched but not well-known area of nutrition is the effect of different foods on our pH balance. Depending on your metabolic dominance, foods can affect you one way and another person the opposite way (Wolcott, 2002). For example, if your metabolism is dominated by oxidation--the speed at which you convert food into energy--foods that would alkalinize your blood pH the most are beef, organ meats, bacon, lentils, butter, heavy cream and salt. On the other end, the foods that would acidify your blood the most are citrus fruits, alcohol, coffee, onions and peppers (Wiley, 1989). If however, your metabolism is dominated by your autonomic nervous system rather than your oxidative system, the opposite is true. Autonomic dominant individuals' blood is acidified most by beef, organ meats, bacon, lentils, butter, heavy cream and salt and alkalinized most by citrus fruits, alcohol, coffee, onions and peppers.

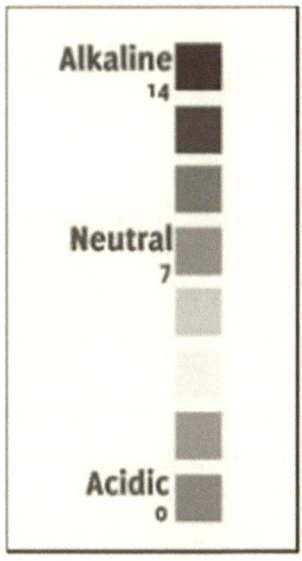

Foods aren't inherently bad or good, as you can see. Whether any food is disastrous or beneficial to your health depends completely on your metabolic type® and your current pH balance or imbalance. It is precisely for this reason that high amounts of meat can be very healthy for certain people, people whose pH is too acidic (a fast oxidizer) or too alkaline (parasympathetic-autonomic dominant). For these folks, meat and heavy fats actually bring their body into a more balanced status. When our bodies are more balanced, not only do we decrease our risk of illness and disease, but we feel more energetic, emotionally balanced, clear-headed, and neither our weight or our food cravings run rampant.

PROTEIN DIGESTIBILITY

Before giving you some generic data on protein digestibility, let me just preface that if you don't have a healthy digestive system, your body isn't going to be absorbing all the vital nutrients it needs from any food source! It is a paradox that digestion improves when your body is balanced, but your body cannot be balanced without good digestion. If you are not eating the right proteins for your body, then you won't be able to achieve good health. So take the following information as a jumping off place for conducting your own experimentation on personal protein digestibility.

Some foods appear to be better sources of protein than they are. If you are interested in how much protein you will absorb from a food (factoring in that you have a healthy digestive system), the NPU (net protein utilization) is a way of measuring how well protein is used by the body.

Eggs have the most ideal proportion of amino acids and dried eggs have the highest NPU value (94%) followed by tempeh (fermented soy) (86%), milk (70-82%), fish (80%), meat (67%), and spirulina, a type of algae (62%). Grains rank similar to spirulina and nuts have a slightly lower NPU than spirulina and grains. When protein quantity is taken into account, we find that spirulina is second only to dried eggs in terms of usable protein as a percentage of the food's composition (http://www.spirulinasource.com/earthfood- ch2a.html). Furthermore, spirulina is very easy to digest and absorb because it has cellulose in its cell walls. This is beneficial for people with intestinal malabsorption. Eggs unfortunately, are a common food allergy (both immediate and delayed).

SOY PROTEIN

Soy protein has recently become very popular as a meat alternative. Many people believe soy to be a great non-meat protein source, if of course they don't have a soy allergy. However, it is contradictory whether soy should make up a significant amount of our diet. There is a fair amount of controversy about whether soy is healthy, or even safe, for humans.

Health Hazards of Soy

Arguments against soy are that the soybean has many toxins which has a negative impact on thyroid hormone production, brain functioning, and reproductive development. These plant toxins also inhibit important enzymes and the mineral zinc (Leduc, 2002). Some enzyme inhibitors in soy block the protein digesting enzyme trypsin, thereby inhibiting protein absorption and digestibility. Hemagglutinin in soy is a clot-promoting substance in soybeans that causes red blood cells to clump together. This can be disastrous to our heart health. Phytic acid, or phytates, present in higher levels in soy than in many other plant foods, block the uptake of minerals such as calcium, magnesium, and especially zinc.

Soy Health Myths

If it's soy you want, your best bet is to eat fermented forms like miso, tempeh and natto. Much of the soy you see in the stores are junk foods disguised as health foods because we've been led to believe that soy is healthy for us. Soy is used to make a lot of different foods including soy hot dogs, ice cream, burgers, cheese, chips, crackers, and cereal. These foods are very processed foods and have had what little nutritional value they started out with removed. They have no place in your diet even if you are vegetarian.

Tofu and soymilk are also processed. The degree of processing depends on the brand. Some companies process more than others. A quick phone call to the company will tell you if the brand you want to drink has minimal processing or not.

Sexual Development Interference

There is some convincing research to support not including soy in your diet at all. Some studies have found that children raised on soy infant formula are at risk of premature sexual development. In fact, soy infant formula was found in one study to be the most significant dietary association of premature sexual development (Random Factoid: chickens raised on soy feed was the runner up). It appears that the phytoestrogens encourage premature puberty onset because the ratio of isoflavones (plant estrogen) to body weight is so high compared to adults. "New Zealand toxicologist Mike Fitzpatrick estimates that an infant exclusively fed soy formula receives the estrogenic equivalent (based on body weight) of at least five birth control pills per day," (Fallon & Enig, 2000).

Estrogenic Effect

Other clinical studies on soy-based infant formula conclude that it is safe and does not adversely affect human growth, reproduction, or development (Merritt & Jenks, 2004). In March 2006, the Center for the Evaluation of Risks to Human Reproduction, a part of the National Institutes of Health, called together a panel of fourteen scientific experts to examine soy formula and genistein, a substance found in soy that has an estrogenic effect. The panel did a thorough review of the existing scientific research to determine if either soy formula or genistein causes problems with reproduction or with development. After its analysis, the panel stated that low to moderate consumption (below 35 milligrams of genistein per kilogram of body weight) does not seem to be harmful. Since infants on soy formula consume only 8 milligrams per kilogram or less of genistein, the panel concluded that there was "little or no reason to be concerned about the safety of genistein for infants using soy formula," (retrieved from http://findarticles.com/p/articles/ mi_m0FDE/is_4_25/ai_n16834303).

While the studies arguing that soy and soy isoflavones are possibly harmful may have a point, many of them are based on animal studies or studies using very small samples. This does not mean their conclusions should be discounted, but further research needs to be done before they hold much credence.

One very good point raised in an article by Mike Fitzpatrick for The Weston Price Foundation is that the soybean has changed very much from what it used to be. Its nutritional content, method of farming, and quantity of consumption is different now.

The Modern Versus Traditional Soybean

The claim that is assumed in scientific literature is that isoflavones have been consumed for thousands of years. This assumption is based on the general presumption that soy consumption was wide-spread in Asia.

Soybean products have been consumed in some parts of Asia for hundreds of years. However, they did not form a significant part of the diet. Also, the traditional soybean was quite different to the soybean we consume today.

The Soybean Has Changed

Glycine soja, the wild soybean, is the species of soybean that was consumed traditionally and is the ancestor of the modern soybean, Glycine max. It is well established that Glycine max is, compositionally, quite different than Glycine soja. While we know from research done sixty years ago that Glycine max contains isoflavones, we do not know that the same can be said for Glycine soja. Glycine max has been cultivated to have more protein and oil as well as to be pest resistant.

It has also been shown that plants such as Glycine max produce phytoestrogens such as the soy isoflavones as a defense mechanism in response to pests. This defense may have served to increase the levels of isoflavones, and other naturally occurring toxins.

It is also well established that different types of Glycine max can contain widely variable levels of isoflavones. Because of this variability, we really don't know if the traditional Asian soybean, Glycine soja, contained very low levels of isoflavones or perhaps none at all.

This more accurate portrayal of soy in the human diet demonstrates that we don't really know whether or not soy or isoflavones are safe. We have been making assumptions based on the traditional soybean, but as you can see, our modern soybean is quite different and hasn't stood the test of time.

Benefits of Soy?

Many people consume soy because they think that it is healthy for them. There are claims that soy is healthy for our hearts, cholesterol, bone density, menopausal symptoms, and may prevent cancers of the breast, uterus and prostate.

In January, 2006 an American Heart Association review (in the journal Circulation) of a decade-long study of soy protein benefits cast doubt on the FDA-allowed "heart healthy" claim for soy protein. What the panel found was that the research does not single out soy isoflavones as preventing heart disease, cancers, or reducing hot flashes on post-menopausal women. What the authors did conclude was that using soy foods such as tofu, soy butter, soy nuts, and some soy burgers to replace high saturated fat and cholesterol animal protein foods "should be beneficial to cardiovascular and overall health because of their high content of polyunsaturated fats, fiber, vitamins, and minerals and low content of saturated fat," (retrieved from http://atvb.ahajournals.org/cgi/content/ full/26/8/1689). As you have already learned by reading this book, saturated fat and cholesterol are not the villains they have been made out to be and instead are absolutely vital to our health.

While we may discover down the road that soy has health benefits for adults, you should proceed with extreme caution. What we do know about soy puts it in a very controversial category at best and an extreme health risk at worst. If you do want to eat or drink it, that is your choice. I recommend listening to your body, as with all foods, and if you notice undesirable symptoms such as gas, bloating, mental fogginess, fatigue, nasal congestion, etc., avoid it for a week or so before trying it again. You may find that you physically and mentally feel better avoiding it. If not, I'd say to consume it with caution.

Better Soy Choices

Fermented soy products such as tempeh (fermented soybean cake), miso (fermented soybean paste), and natto (fermented soybeans) may be healthier, since the fermentation process neutralizes toxins such as phytic acid and enzyme inhibitors (retrieved from www.westonaprice.org/The-Ploy-of-Soy.html). Also, as is true of all foods, quality makes a big difference when it comes to the health properties of soy. Buy soy products that are non-GMO (genetically modified).

So, stick to tempeh, miso, soymilk without a lot of added sweeteners, and non-GMO (genetically modified) tofu. Unless you eat hot dogs, chips, and other junk foods, it is not healthier to eat the soy alternatives just because they are made with soy!

OTHER NON-ANIMAL PROTEIN

Other rich sources of non-animal protein include legumes, nuts, seeds, yeast, and freshwater algae. Food yeasts such as "nutritional yeast" and "brewer's yeast" are extremely nutritious additions to foods such as soups, stews, sauces, dips, casseroles, breads and even popcorn. Most yeasts get about fifty percent of their calories from protein (retrieved from http://www.happycow.net).

Hemp Protein

Hemp seeds are incredibly nutritious. They contain a good amount of balanced protein, almost 35 grams per 100 grams of seeds, and are also high in both Omega-3 and Omega-6 fatty acids. Hemp seeds actually have the best ratio compared to other foods of these two essential fatty acids. These benefits along with their high antioxidant, vitamin and mineral content make hemp seeds a great food to include in your diet.

VEGETARIANS AND PROTEIN

I can't write a chapter about protein without a section on vegetarianism. While I think their hearts are in the right place, most people's bodies will not function optimally on a strict vegetarian diet (i.e., excluding foods that are of animal origin including meat, fish, poultry, eggs, dairy, gelatin, honey, etc.). Lacto-vegetarians include milk and milk products but still exclude all other animal-derived foods. Lacto-ovu-vegetarians eat milk and milk products and eggs, but still exclude other animal-derived foods (Whitney & Rolfes, 2002). Lacto-vegetarians and lacto-ovu-vegetarians are exposed to more of the valuable nutrients found in animal products and therefore won't have as many gaps in their diet as strict vegetarians or vegans.

As far as protein is concerned, I mentioned earlier that protein is easy to come by and vegetarians can get protein from nuts and seeds, grains, milk and other dairy products. They can also obtain protein from pulses--such as lentils and beans, vegetables, and mycoprotein (protein-rich foodstuff made from processed, edible fungus—the leading brand is called Quorn and can be found at http://www.quorn.us). Most of these non-animal sources of protein do not have purines (a special component in some proteins that aids in metabolism). Certain people require more purines in their diet and would suffer on a vegetarian diet lacking this important nutrient.

VEGETARIANS AND MINERALS

Our bodies handle minerals such as zinc and iron very carefully and can adjust how much we store. In a perfect world, vegetarians generally are not at increased risk of being iron or zinc deficient since their bodies adapt to a meat-free diet by absorbing these minerals more efficiently (Whitney & Rolfes, 2002). However, we don't live in a perfect world and our bodies are exposed to a number of factors that increase our need for iron and zinc (environmental toxins, diuretics, absorption problems, nutrient competition from plant-based foods). Individuals that require more of these minerals will fall short on a vegetarian diet.

VEGETARIANS AND B12

An obvious sign that humans are intended to eat animals is shown by Vitamin B12. Vitamin B12 is only found in significant, absorbable form in animal-derived foods. Foods that are fortified such as breads, cereals, and soy milk supply part of a vegetarian's B12 requirement, but a supplement is absolutely recommended to avoid neurological issues from developing from lack of this important vitamin (retrieved from http://www.medicalnewstoday.com/ articles/8749.php).

PROTEIN AND CALCIUM: WHAT IS GOING ON?

The relationship between protein, calcium, and bone density is controversial. Some research demonstrates that as protein intake increases, calcium stores from bones decrease despite high calcium supplementation. Other research demonstrates that as long as sufficient fruits, vegetables, quality fats, and calcium are present in the diet, a high protein diet does not cause a net loss of calcium from our bones. There are strong arguments on both sides making this one of the largest continued controversies in nutrition.

After reviewing a large volume of scientific research, it appears that when there is substantial calcium in the diet (approximately 1,000-1,500 mg of calcium per day), protein helps calcium build stronger bones. However, if calcium intake is low, protein actually increases bone loss because it increases urinary loss of calcium (Heaney, 2002). Normally, protein works with calcium to build bones and heal bones. If either one is too low, our bone health suffers. If calcium intake is sufficient but protein intake isn't, the research suggests that we don't build as much bone density as we do when both calcium and protein intake is higher. Because different metabolic types® handle both calcium and protein differently, the results of these studies cannot be generalized to everyone. In fact, part of the reason there is conflicting scientific data is because they aren't taking biochemical individuality into account when they conduct their research! It is highly recommended that you discover your metabolic type® so you can tailor your protein and calcium needs.

This is good news for individuals who find they do better with a bit more protein in their diets. As long as you get plenty of calcium, eat good healthy fats and whole foods rich in nutrition, and don't go overboard with protein, you are not at increased risk for osteoporosis. Too much protein, however, can be bad for your bones if your metabolic type® requires less protein.

In the Nurses' Health Study of 1980, for example, over 85,000 women contributed to the findings that women who ate more than 95 grams of protein a day were 20 percent more likely to have broken a wrist over a 12-year period when compared to those who ate an average amount of protein (less than 68 grams a day). The quality of the protein they ate was not specified (retrieved from http:// www.ncbi.nlm.nih.gov/sites/entrez?cmd=Retrieve&db=PubMed&li st_uids=8610662&dopt=AbstractPlus).

Other studies have found similar patterns of increased risk of fractures when protein intake is high. Remember though, that research studies don't account for biochemical individuality and so it is impossible to draw a conclusion that is going to fit every person.

PROTEIN AND MINERAL ABSORPTION WITHIN DIFFERENT METABOLIC TYPES®

Since our bodies handle nutrients differently, it is important to consider how different answers can be given within research studies. Taking the research on wrist fractures and high protein intake, the results could have been completely different depending on if the researchers had controlled for metabolic type®. For example, calcium is needed in higher amounts in protein type metabolic types® (fast oxidizers and parasympathetics) but these types also need relatively more protein and fat than their metabolic counterparts. A likely scenario is that wrist fractures were more common in those individuals whose metabolic types® require less protein (carb types: sympathetic dominants or slow oxidizers). These are the kinds of questions that don't get addressed in most mainstream research, but entirely clouds how applicable the results of the study are!

While future research may improve on the concept of bioindividuality, for now, it is wise to eat right for your metabolic type® since that is associated with the best overall health benefits.

BONES AND FLUORIDE

An important side note regarding bone health is that sodium fluoride added to drinking water is not good for building strong, sturdy bones. It causes an apparent increase in bone mass, but the bone structure is abnormal and weak. Recent studies indicate that hip fractures are more common in areas where water is fluoridated.

Find out if your water is fluoridated and if it is; strongly consider a filtration system for your home. Drinking bottled water only protects you to a point. We absorb fluoride and other minerals through our skin, so every time you shower, wash your face, do the dishes, or brush your teeth, you are being exposed to more and more fluoride. You can individually purchase shower and faucet filters if it is not within your

117

budget to install a home filtration unit. These are great for reducing your exposure to all sorts of harmful elements (like chlorine) in addition to fluoride.

CHOOSING QUALITY PROTEIN

1. When I eat protein this week, I will write down which types my body feels the best with afterward. I will try at least two different protein sources.

2. I will eat a higher amount of unprocessed protein (beef vs. lunchmeat, tempeh vs. tofu) and observe if I notice a difference in how I feel and how much energy I have.

3. I will eat two meals this week that have animal sources of protein and two meals with vegetable sources of protein and observe if I notice a difference in how I feel and how much energy I have.

Chapter 8

Metabolism

Metabolism is talked about in such a way these days that you'd think it were the Holy Grail: something we are seeking and yet can't seem to find. In truth, metabolism is happening inside you every second of every day. Metabolism is the total of all the chemical reactions that go on in living cells (the body). At any given point, our bodies are doing a variety of tasks that require chemical reactions and so our metabolic wheels are constantly turning. Energy metabolism pertains to the way the body obtains and spends the energy from food. This will be what we focus on in this chapter.

What people seem most interested in is speeding up their metabolism so they can either lose weight, eat more, or both. There are ways of increasing your metabolism, which I will discuss in this chapter. What is more important than a fast metabolism, though, is a healthy metabolism. Poor nutrition, lack of sleep, stress and lack of physical activity are detrimental to a healthy metabolism. Every step that you take towards improving your total health will in turn help your metabolism. To understand this more clearly, let's take a look at the different components of our metabolism.

FACTORS THAT INCREASE METABOLISM

Having a fast metabolism is not as important as having a healthy metabolism. Bear in mind that getting plenty of quality sleep, managing stress, regular physical activity, staying hydrated and eating healthy foods at regular intervals daily are essential to a healthy metabolism. If you are already doing these things, here are some additional suggestions for healthily speeding up your metabolism. Take them with a grain of salt: everyone is different and therefore changes should be made one at a time and cautiously so that you can better observe how your unique body chemistry is handling the change.

- Eat the right balance of protein, fat and carbs for your body. The brain uses two-thirds (65%) of total glucose/day or approximately 400-600 calories! (Castner, 2001). Carbohydrates are an obvious source of glucose, but your body can make all the glucose/ketones you need from fat and protein. This may work much better for you if you are sensitive to starches such as grains or vegetables and fruits that are higher in sugar (e.g., beets, dates). Choosing vegetables and fruits and combining them with quality proteins and fats, provides glucose for your brain and also keeps your blood sugar balanced.

- Strength training is a key method for boosting one's metabolism. For every pound of muscle built, our Basal Metabolic Rate (BMR) increases up to 50 kcals/day and fat burning by as much as 62%!

- Cardiovascular exercise is a great way to boost EEPA metabolism (Energy Expended from Physical Activity). The longer that you exercise, the more total calories you burn in a day. Higher intensity (harder or faster) cardio will burn more calories than slow, steady exercise as long as the intensity doesn't cause you to end the exercise session too early. If you work too hard and run out of breath so that you have to stop, the exercise no longer qualifies as aerobic ("with oxygen") and the total calories burned may not be enough to significantly boost your EEPA. However, less intense cardiovascular exercise is still very beneficial and may be superior when it comes to personal enjoyment and sticking with it long-term.

- Essential fatty acids found in flax oil, olive oil, nuts and seeds also stimulate metabolism because the body converts them to prostaglandins. These prostaglandins help increase metabolism. (Caution: see Chapter 6 on Fats to learn about oxidization of these delicate fats).

- Vitamin B6 and the minerals manganese and zinc help convert fats to prostaglandins.

- Eat at regular intervals and do NOT skip meals. Many studies have confirmed that people who eat 4-6 meals per day have less body fat than those who eat 2-3 meals per day even though both groups ate the same amount of calories! The frequency of meals increases TEF (Thermic Effect of Food).

- Skipping meals or snacking on high sugared foods increases your body's production of insulin and leads to increased fat storage as well as boosts your chances of overeating when you do eat. Furthermore, your body's fat cells can actually adapt to a pattern of eating large, infrequent meals by becoming more efficient at storing fat! To help keep your insulin balanced and your metabolism happy, eat healthy snacks between meals such as nuts, seeds, meats, cheeses, or beans with veggies or whole grains.

- Capsaicin (the nutrient that makes peppers hot) increases enzymes responsible for fat metabolism in the liver.

- Coconut oil stimulates the thyroid gland (the main metabolism gland).

METABOLISM BASICS

The body converts food into a usable form of energy: calories. Every food provides a certain amount of energy or calories. Calories are a measure of the amount of energy a food can provide. A common abbreviation for calories is kcals (since one calorie is really 1,000 calories, but in the United States it is simplified). Carbohydrates have 4.1 kcals per gram and proteins provide 4.3. Fats have kcals per gram, more than twice the energy per gram than both carbohydrates and proteins (Sharkey, 2002).

When we take in more energy (calories) than our bodies can use, or we take in the wrong nutrients for our body, the excess energy is stored as fat. Fat is so important for good health that our bodies can make it from any food: carbs, protein, sugar--you name it! Any nutrient in excess is stored as fat. Carbohydrates eaten in excess are first stored in our muscles and liver as muscle glycogen and liver glycogen (as mentioned in Chapter 5). We cannot store protein, so the excess is converted and stored as fat. Excess fat is always stored as fat.

It is generally agreed that of the three nutrients, fat is usually the most efficiently stored as fat. The body has to work harder and expend more calories to break protein and carbohydrates down into a form that can be stored as fat. This is why most diets tell you to eat less fat. The body only has to use five percent of its energy to store fat as fat, whereas converting carbohydrates into a form that can be stored as fat requires around twenty-five percent. When excess calories are eaten, the body will first use carbs and protein for energy and other body functions like building muscle, and then the excess gets stored as fat. Fat has its important roles to serve as well, but it is the most efficient of the three to be stored as fat.

As with every bodily function, there are many variations to each rule. Some people need considerably more fat in their diets to be healthy and have a healthy metabolism. The above generalizations about fat storage can be misconstrued. Fat is definitely not the enemy. Yes, for some people, if they eat too much fat, it will make them fat, but the same can be said for protein and carbohydrates.

Human metabolism is more complicated than previously thought. Clearly, it doesn't just boil down to counting calories. All calories are not handled equally. The magic link appears to be with controlling

123

insulin levels, rather than keeping calories low.

ENZYME LEVELS GIVE US A CLUE

Enzymatically, the human body has many more enzymes for digesting protein and fat than carbohydrates. Proteolytic enzymes (enzymes for breaking down protein) can break down up to 300 grams of protein per hour. Lipolytic enzymes (enzymes for breaking down fats) can break down up to 175 grams of fat per hour.

Compare that to amylolytic enzymes which only break down up to 300 grams of carbohydrates per day and it becomes clear which nutrients we should consume more than others. We are much more enzymatically geared to consume protein and fat. Like everything else, there is variation from person to person. At risk of sounding like a broken record, it really is in your best interest to find out your metabolic type® and eat accordingly. Knowing as much as you can about your metabolic individuality will help ensure that you are eating the right amounts of protein, fat, and carbs to keep your insulin levels (and your waistline) in check.

COMPONENTS OF METABOLISM

Basal Metabolic Rate (BMR or REE) is the energy expended to maintain life (breathing, heartbeat, etc.). These vital functions re-quire a great deal of energy even though we do them unconsciously. BMR accounts for 65% of all our calories burned!

Energy Expended from Physical Activity (EEPA) accounts for 20-40% of calories burned per day. This is a huge variance and helps to ex-plain why exercise plays such a large part in weight loss by increasing metabolism.

Thermic Effect of Food (TEF) is the energy expended for digestion, absorption of nutrients, etc., and accounts for roughly 10% of our total energy output. Generally, higher carbohydrate meals have a higher

Thermic effect than high fat meals. There is so much variance between people and their TEF that this component isn't even used to calculate total energy output. Even so, it is important to mention that it plays a role (in some people, the role is bigger than in others) in metabolism.

Adaptive Thermogenesis refers to the changes in energy expenditure that accompany changes in the environment such as cold weather versus warm weather, but also to physiological events such as changes in hormonal levels and injuries (Castner, 2001). Because this metabolic factor is so variable from person to person, like TEF, it is not often used when calculating total energy output.

FACTORS THAT DECREASE METABOLISM

- Snacking on high sugared foods throughout the day. Also eating or drinking sweets before exercise reduces weight loss (increases insulin and fat storage).
- Eating overly large meals leads to an increase in fat storage, slows BMR and tricks the body into starvation mode.
- Fasting. When we don't eat, our metabolism slows down, less fat is burned, and our appetite is decreased.

- The wrong macronutrient ratios! Not getting the right mixture of proteins, fats and carbs leads to a sluggish metabolism. Without the right fuel, your body will not operate optimally, build and maintain muscle or burn fat adequately.

- Age. Metabolism will decrease unless muscle is maintained through strength training.
- Alcohol decreases metabolism and impairs the liver's ability to metabolize fats.

Gary Taubes' book *Good Calories, Bad Calories* is full of research over the past one hundred years linking obesity to a problem with metabolism. Specifically, many studies show that on a diet low in carbohydrates, the body's ability to burn fat improves tremendously.

People could eat fat and protein to their heart's content and still lose weight, but when carbohydrates were incorporated, their insulin levels increased and so did their waistlines. Clearly, there is a great deal of hormonal influence on weight loss. Time to retire the calorie counting and focus on eating to support total health!

METABOLIC SUPPLEMENTS

- Drugs such as Orlistat (Xenical) are weight loss pills that can inhibit the absorption of dietary fats by blocking the enzymes that break down fat in our bodies, allowing around 30% of fat to pass through the gut undigested and therefore help reduce excess body fat in obese people. Xenical also impedes absorption of fat soluble vitamins and so should be used with caution and under the care of a physician. Another popular weight loss pill is Sibutramine (Meridia) which works differently than Xenical. It works on the part of your brain that controls hunger and is supposed to help you feel full. Its side effects can be anything from dizziness, headaches, pounding heart rate and nausea to seizures, numbness/tingling of hands or feet, to, ironically, increased appetite (Castner, 2001). In my opinion, weight loss pills should never be used. They introduce more problems than they help and do not support long-term health or weight loss.

- Chromium supplements alone do not help increase metabolism or fat loss or muscle gain, but it is important to get enough chromium to meet the body's needs. Chromium is important for balancing insulin and assisting in fat metabolism. Supplements are helpful for correcting a deficiency.

- Ma Huang (Ephedra) is a central nervous system stimulant. When taken alone, Ma Huang doesn't help you lose weight. When combined with caffeine and a calorie restricted diet, studies found that Ma Huang did help weight loss but it had adverse side effects such as increased heart rate and blood pressure and can be lethal if taken by those with heart ailments, high blood pressure, thyroid conditions or diabetes.

CALCULATING YOUR DAILY CALORIC INTAKE

Unless you go to a clinic and are hooked up to a machine for twenty-four hours or more so that your oxygen intake can be measured, you will not know exactly how many calories you require per day to maintain your weight, lose weight, or gain weight.

However, you can estimate your total energy expenditure. There are many formulas available. I recommend trying several and take the average number as your estimated daily caloric expenditure. Using caloric expenditure should only be used in conjunction with metabolic typing® since eating the right foods for your body is step number one toward achieving a healthy weight.

Basal Metabolic Rate

Calculate BMR using the Harris-Benedict Equation (even though it has been found to overestimate BMR by 7-24%). As I mentioned, none of the formulas are perfect because there are so many factors to account for, but this one is better than most.

Step 1: Take your weight in pounds and divide by 2.2 to get kilograms.

Step 2: Take your height in inches (5 feet=60 inches) and multiply by 2.54 to get centimeters.

Step 3: Take these numbers that you get and plug them into the following equation:

Women: BMR (kcal) = 655 + 9.56(weight in kg) + 1.85(height in cm) - 4.68(age)

Men: BMR (kcal) = 66.5 + 13.7(weight in kg) + 5.0(height in cm) −

6.78(age)

For obese individuals (those with a BMI over 30), it is best to use the following formula for calculating basal metabolic rate:

(Actual Body Weight – Ideal Body Weight) x .25 + Ideal Body Weight
Physical Activity Factor

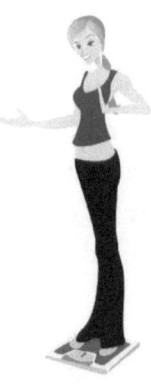

Now that you have an estimated BMR, the next step is to estimate how much energy you expend daily with physical activity. Choose from the options below and multiply your BMR by the number that corresponds best with your current activity level:

Sedentary (no exercise) =1.0-1.2
Slight Physical Activity (<60 min of cardio/week)=1.2-1.4
Moderate Physical Activity (<180 min cardio/week)=1.4-1.6
Heavy Physical Activity (>180 min cardio & strength training) =1.6-1.8
Endurance Exercise (>420 min cardio + 150 min strength training) =1.8-2.0

Once you have multiplied your BMR with the Physical Activity Factor that best describes your activity pattern, this number is your estimated daily caloric intake requirement. This number by itself does not mean anything. If you choose to monitor your caloric intake (what you eat each day) as well as your caloric output (the calories you burn with exercise), then you can see how you are doing with balancing your energy needs. If you wish to gain or lose weight, you will need to adjust both your food intake and your exercise output.

More on this later!

HEALTHY METABOLISM PLAN

Now that you know the basics of metabolism and have an estimate for how many calories you burn in a day, you can start making more educated decisions about your lifestyle choices. Here are some suggestions for you to try. You will know which ones are working for you by the changes you see in your energy level, mood, and body weight. Try one suggestion at a time so you can better gauge its effects on your unique body chemistry.

- Eat small meals throughout the day rather than fewer large meals. To help you stay satisfied between meals, choose a mixture of protein, fat and carbohydrate with each small meal.

- Pay attention to serving sizes. Because you will be eating more frequently, you may need to eat less at each meal. Rate your hunger both at the start and end of your small meal. On a scale of 1-10, 1 being famished and 10 being stuffed, eat before your hunger level is 1 or 2 and stop eating when it reaches 7 or 8.

- Eat a variety of foods throughout the day. Different foods offer different vitamins and minerals so it is good to eat a variety of colors, textures, and tastes. However, with each small meal, select only two to three different foods. Studies do show that having too many food choices at each meal tends to lead to overeating and weight gain (Roizen & Oz, 2006).

- Get tested for food allergies. When you consume foods that you are allergic to, you disrupt your metabolic system (and therefore every other system in your body!).

- Strength train every week—three days are optimal, but one or two is better than zero!

- Integrate some higher intensity bursts into your cardio session. Try speeding up for 15-30 seconds every five minutes.

- Use quality fats such as raw butter, coconut oil, flax, and olive oil rather than hydrogenated oils and margarines.

- Eat foods rich in zinc, manganese, and Vitamin B6. Dark green leafy vegetables such as kale, chard, spinach, mustard/turnip/beet greens are high in zinc and manganese. Potatoes, chicken breast, soy, bananas, and beans are great sources of B6. (Remember that eating the right foods for your metabolic type® is much more essential to a healthy metabolism than single vitamin or mineral supplementation.)

You now have a number of tools for improving your metabolic health. As I mentioned, start with one suggestion at a time and notice the improvements. If you are interested in weight loss or are just curious how close your current calorie intake matches the estimated daily calorie requirements that we figured out earlier, keep a food journal for three days (to get an average). You can figure out what your current caloric intake is by using a helpful calorie counting website like www.fitday.com, a book of foods and their caloric amounts like Corinne Netzer's Complete Book of Food Counts, or an online database like the USDA National Nutrient Database (http://www.nal.usda.gov/fnic/foodcomp/search/). At the very least, this will be an educational experience for you and at best, it will awaken and motivate you toward a healthier diet, improved energy, and the validation that you took charge of your health.

CHOOSING A HEALTHY METABOLISM

1. I will choose one item on the "Healthy Metabolism Plan" and stick to it for a minimum of two days.

2. I will choose one dietary item and one activity on the "Healthy Metabolism Plan" and stick to it for a minimum of one week.

3. I will calculate my estimated daily caloric intake and observe how well I seem to metabolize different nutrients. I will choose one dietary item and one activity on the "Healthy Metabolism Plan" and stick to it for a minimum of one month.

Chapter 9

Grocery Shopping

Weekly grocery shopping is an essential component to building and maintaining your healthy lifestyle. Without the proper ingredients to put together healthy meals and snacks, your segue into a healthier lifestyle won't get very far! Rather than looking at weekly trips to the grocery store as tedious annoyances, look at it like this: if there are no groceries in the house, you don't have food to eat just like if you don't have toilet paper in the bathroom...well, you get the picture. Regardless of its convenience, grocery shopping needs to be done. If you have the resources to have someone do it for you, great, but most of us don't. Let's accept it and move past "whether it needs to be done or not" to "how best to go about it."

GROCERY SHOPPING 101

When going to a place where you are surrounded by food temptations, ingenious marketing, and "Buy 4 get 8 Free!" deals, you must have a plan to keep you on track. Here are some basics that everyone should know and follow:

1. Make a grocery list at home.

2. Stick to your grocery list.

These really are the only two rules that are essential to successful grocery shopping. The other minor detail is of course, having a comprehensive shopping list. You can go about this in several ways.

1. Go through your fridge and cupboards every week and write

down what you are out of that you want to eat the following week.

2. Keep a shopping template to save time (you will still occasionally need to do the old fridge and cupboard rummaging).

If you are grocery shopping for the first time, start out with a short grocery list and familiarize yourself with the store. Don't be afraid to ask where things are. If you have to wander the aisles looking for everything, it can take a long time. Do yourself a favor and ask for help and then remember where things are. Pretty soon, you will have a clear layout of the store and your shopping trips will become much faster.

ANATOMY OF A GROCERY STORE

With few exceptions, most of the "real food" in most grocery stores is on the outer perimeter of the store and not the aisles in between. This is where you will find the fresh foods that haven't been overly processed. If you do most of your shopping from the perimeter, chances are that you'll be eating healthier by default. You'll also save time and money since packaging and marketing is expensive and neither are in abundance on fresh fruits, vegetables, meats, and cheeses.

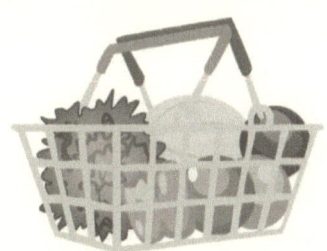

Limit your shopping in the center aisles that contain chips, cookies, sodas, frozen dinners, canned fruits and veggies, fruit cocktails, etc. If there are certain things you really want to buy and they don't conflict with your personal health goal, then put them on your list and stick to those items only. It is easy to get distracted in the store, especially if you are hungry, so I can't emphasize enough how important it is to stick to your list!

The Beginning Shopper

Some good shopping basics will help you to keep it simple.

- Write a grocery list based on things you know you will eat in the next week.
- Don't buy foods that you only eat on occasion because the chances are high that you won't get to it before it goes bad and you will waste both time and money.
- Pick your favorite healthy foods and make your best guess as to how much to get. You will quickly learn how much of certain foods to buy, but for now, underestimate.

Here is a sample grocery list for a single person for one week:

- 2 bunches lettuce/spinach or 2 bags salad mix
- Balsamic vinegar
- 2 bunches cauliflower
- 1 bunch carrots
- 1 jar of almond or peanut butter
- 1 jar fruit spread
- 1 loaf gluten free bread
- 1 package chicken breasts or thighs (you can freeze them and portion them out for the week)
- 2 fish fillets and/or beef roast
- 8 medium to large shiitake mushrooms
- ½ gallon raw milk or almond milk
- ½ dozen eggs
- 1 container whole oats and/or chia seeds
- 7 apples
- 7 yogurts
- 1 bag nuts

With this list, there are snack options for the whole week (celery, carrots, apples, yogurt and nuts) and the makings for breakfasts (oatmeal or chia porridge and eggs/veggie scramble), lunches and dinners (chicken/fish/beef, cauliflower and salad OR salad topped with egg, chicken, fish or beef roast OR vegetarian dinner with shiitake mushrooms, eggs, and veggies or almond butter and jelly sandwiches). This list is very simple and doesn't add for much food variety, but it is great if you are just starting out with cooking and shopping for yourself. Get comfortable with the process first and then let your creativity grow!

*Note: This grocery list is for people who do not feel their best when consuming meat often or starch often. If your body does best consuming meat frequently and/or needs more starch, adjust accordingly.

SHOPPING TIPS FOR FAMILIES

When shopping for more than one person, things can get a lot more complicated if each person has a different set of dietary needs. If everyone in the family thrives on the same foods, then just buy more of each item. If there are special dietary considerations, there are strategies for making shopping simpler. For example, if someone in your household is vegetarian, it is easiest to prepare vegetarian dishes and then serve some meat on the side if desired. If a family member is allergic/intolerant to wheat, you can still make spaghetti or lasagna but use spaghetti squash, shirataki noodles, or gluten-free noodles instead of wheat. Using these substitutions will broaden your food horizon and make shopping and cooking easier. Cooking two separate meals is hard work.

Unfortunately, if your and your family's dietary choices are opposite of each other, cooking totally separate meals may be unavoidable. In this situation, making separate shopping lists makes sense.

135

Organizing shopping according to themed meal nights can save you time and brain power—and it can give everyone some consistency to look forward to. For example, Monday nights can be shredded chicken taco night with salad and beans on the side; Tuesday can be fish, asparagus, and a salad; and maybe Wednesday is leftovers night. Having this kind of meal organization makes grocery shopping very straightforward and it will cut down the time you spend staring blankly in the fridge or cupboards. Give it a try and see how it works for you

Getting Kids Involved

If you grocery shop with your kids, decide ahead of time to stick to your grocery list. Ask family members ahead of time for input on what foods they would like you to buy or what they'd like to eat for themed meal nights. This is a great way to get other family members involved in meal planning and grocery shopping. If you bring your kid(s) to the grocery store with you, give them an age-appropriate job to do like crossing items off the list as you buy them, helping you put fruits and veggies into bags, or picking out yogurt flavors.

Kids can even help in the kitchen if they are given tasks that match their skill level for their age. Food prep takes most of the time for many meals, so ask your kids to help wash vegetables, peel or cut them (suggested for kids age eight and up), help make the salad, set the table, or pour water into glasses for everyone. At first, you will probably spend more time teaching your kids how to help in the kitchen, but once they get the hang of it, their help will save you time and they will feel like they were part of the process.

SHOPPING TIPS FOR SINGLES

The biggest hurdle for singles when it comes to grocery shopping is talking yourself out of how much of a waste of time it is to cook for just one person. It is not a waste of time to nourish yourself! It is true that cooking for someone else and having them praise your culinary genius is rewarding. If this is very important to you, have friends and family over often and cook for them. They will love this!

You can also bring leftovers in to work with you the next day for your lunch and possibly share them with a coworker or bring them to a friend's house for dinner the following night. The beauty of cooking for one is that you are likely to have leftovers and therefore won't have to cook for every meal. Use the sample shopping list from above as a template and get shopping!

GROCERY SHOPPING CHECKLIST

1. Pick a shopping day (at least once per week) and try to stick to it.

2. Always go to the store with a grocery list.

3. Make a list based on recipes you plan on preparing that week (you can use meal planning websites, phone apps, or just write out your own weekly meal plan).

4. Make a list based on the different food groups so you are assured a variety of healthy foods at home. If you take the test to learn your metabolic type®, you will be given a list of foods already separated into categories: Pick your favorites from each section and viola— you have your grocery list!

5. Try to avoid aisles that you know have danger foods in them to help resist temptation.

6. Don't go to the grocery store hungry. You will be more likely to give in to cravings.

7. Shop from your list, saving perishables until last. And remember, stick to your list!

ADDITIONAL SHOPPING GUIDE TIPS

- Read food labels and compare brands to see which ones are healthier! See Brand Suggestion table below.

- Don't buy brands that have hydrogenated oil or trans fats (read ingredients!)

- Look for carbs with at least two grams of fiber.

- Limit added sugar (compare total carbs to sugar and fiber). Read ingredients! Avoid high fructose corn syrup, sugar, sucrose, and even honey in the first few ingredients.

- Choose local foods whenever possible (unless you know that the quality of food near you is poor). This goes for veggies, fruits, dairy, meat, eggs, etc. Local foods tend to be fresher and less expensive.

- Choose whole dairy products. Yes, they are higher in fat, but they are less processed and contain the percentages of fat, protein and carbohydrate that nature intended.

- To find the percentage of carb, fat, and protein in a food, multiply grams of either carb or protein by 4 and then divide into "total calories." Multiply by 100. For fat you would multiply by 9, but food labels already tell you calories from fat.

- Don't buy more than you need or think you will use just because it's on sale.

REBECCA'S BRAND SUGGESTIONS*

Meats: Local grass-fed, Nihman Ranch, Fulton Valley, Shelton, Diestel, U.S. Wellness, Applegate Farms, Organic Prairie

Nut Butters: Maranatha, Adam's, Laura Scudder's, local & organic brands (like Santa Cruz Organics!)

Jams & Jellies: Crofter's Organics, Santa Cruz Organics, Smuckers Simply Fruit or Trader Joe's Organic Spreadable Fruit

Frozen Foods: Organic veggies (no salt added) & organic fruits

Juices: Santa Cruz Organic, R.W. Knudsen, Walnut Acres, V8 (low sodium is better), Northland, Ocean Spray 100% Juice, & TJ's

Yogurt: White Mountain, Strauss Family Creamery, Clover, Brown Cow, Nancy's, Trader Joe's Organic, and Mountain High (avoid yogurts w/ aspartame and sucralose; choose full-fat yogurts with lower sugar & active cultures). Try plain organic yogurt and add a small amount of maple syrup, fresh fruit or a teaspoon of spreadable fruit and/or some walnuts. Yum!

Chips: Jackson's Honest, Epic Pork Rinds, Garden of Eatin'

Cereals: Enjoy Life, Barbara's, Arrowhead Mills Organic, Nature's Path Mesa Sunrise

Breads/bagels/muffins: Food for Life, Ezekiel, Manna, (look for "gluten-free" "sprouted", low or no added sugar, and no hydrogenated or partially hydrogenated oils)

Crackers: Simply Mills, Mary's Gone Crackers

Cookies: Simply Mills, Newman's Own

Ice Cream: Three Twins, Strauss Family Creamery, Julie's Organics, Breyer's, Haagen Daaz Five, Ruby's Rockets, Dreyer's Whole Fruit Pops (except for the no sugar added ones which have aspartame)

*This list is by no means exhaustive, so I encourage you to read labels and keep adding to this list!

*Brands vary depending on location—visit your local health food store to find out.

READING FOOD LABELS

First, I would suggest that the majority of the foods you buy not be in a package with a food label (fresh fruits, veggies, etc.). For those foods that do have a nutritional facts section, it is important that you know how to read it. With all the fancy marketing, labeling regulations and health claims on foods, you almost need to take a language course in "label-ese." After reading this section, you will have a clear understanding of the nutrition facts panel as well as some of the more obscure facets of food labels. The FDA's guide to reading food labels is thorough and visually comprehensive so I have included it here:

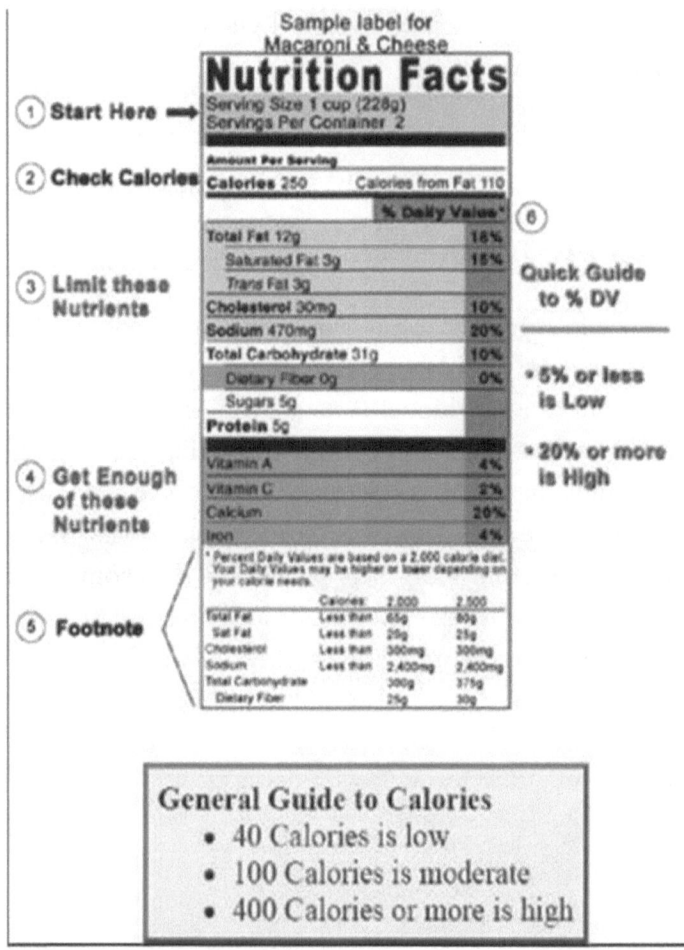

Sample label for
Macaroni & Cheese

Nutrition Facts

(1) **Start Here** ➡ Serving Size 1 cup (228g)
Servings Per Container 2

Amount Per Serving

Calories 250   Calories from Fat 110

(2) **Check Calories**

	% Daily Value*
Total Fat 12g	18%
Saturated Fat 3g	15%
Trans Fat 3g	
Cholesterol 30mg	10%
Sodium 470mg	20%
Total Carbohydrate 31g	10%
Dietary Fiber 0g	0%
Sugars 5g	
Protein 5g	

(3) **Limit these Nutrients**

(4) **Get Enough of these Nutrients**

Vitamin A	4%
Vitamin C	2%
Calcium	20%
Iron	4%

* Percent Daily Values are based on a 2,000 calorie diet. Your Daily Values may be higher or lower depending on your calorie needs.

(5) **Footnote**

	Calories:	2,000	2,500
Total Fat	Less than	65g	80g
Sat Fat	Less than	20g	25g
Cholesterol	Less than	300mg	300mg
Sodium	Less than	2,400mg	2,400mg
Total Carbohydrate		300g	375g
Dietary Fiber		25g	30g

(6) **Quick Guide to % DV**

• **5% or less is Low**

• **20% or more is High**

General Guide to Calories
- 40 Calories is low
- 100 Calories is moderate
- 400 Calories or more is high

There are other aspects to food labels that are not as easy to decipher, but are just as important. These include what "whole grain" really means, how trans fats sneak their way under the label radar, and how both meat and dairy can appear on a label to be a lot lower in fat than they actually are.

WHOLE GRAIN

I suggest eating gluten-free grains. If a label says "made with whole grain," this just means that there is some undefined amount of whole grain in the item. It could be a little or a lot. To avoid having to decipher how much is whole grain, look for the words "100% whole grain" or read the ingredient list (all of the grains should say "whole"). Don't be fooled by "multigrain" either. This just means that a mixture of grains were used to make the food but it may very well be refined mixed grains and therefore less nutritious than just one type of "whole" grain.

Sprouted whole grains are an even better choice since the sprouting process reduces certain mineral binding substances.

FAT FREE/CALORIE FREE/TRANS FAT FREE

If there is a half gram or less of either fat or trans fats per serving, the food label can legally say that it is "non-fat" or "no trans fats." You can read the ingredient list to get a better idea if a food is truly free of fat and/or trans fats.

I don't recommend buying fat-free foods. Fat is a vital nutrient that we all require to be healthy. If you are trying to reduce fat in your diet, eat smaller portions of full-fat foods. No one needs trans fats, however, so read labels carefully to avoid accidentally eating them.

For calories, if a serving size has five calories or less, it can be called "calorie free." Five calories isn't much, but remember that this is just for one serving and many of us eat more than one, especially if we think it is calorie free!

MEAT AND DAIRY LABELING

Look for 100% grass-fed and finished. Beyond that, here is some useful label information on the fat content. I am not advocating buying low fat or non-fat products. If, however, your body does better with less fat, this information is critical to your success and in general, it is just good information to have.

Whereas the FDA labels fat content by calories, the USDA is in charge of regulating meat and dairy and they label fat content by volume or weight instead. For example, if you buy ground beef that says "93% lean," this means that only 7% of its weight is from fat—but it actually has 44% of its calories from fat.

For dairy, look for organic, raw, grass-fed, and non-homogenized. For fat content, one percent milk has 18% of fat by calories; two percent has 36%, and whole milk has 49%. Do yourself a favor: if you want to know how much fat a serving of meat or dairy has, look at the nutrition facts label. Take the "calories from fat" and divide that number into the "total calories per serving."

For example, using our 93% lean ground beef we have 160 calories per serving and 70 calories from fat which, when we divide one by the other, gives us about 44% calories from fat. 70 cals from fat/160 cals per serving=.4375 x 100= 44% calories from fat.

Quick Shopping Guide for Lower Fat Meat

If a 3.5 ounce serving of beef has less than 5 grams of fat, less than 2 grams saturated fat and less than 95 mg of cholesterol, it is considered "extra lean" (www.lowfatcooking.about.com).

The following cuts of meat are extra lean:

- Eye Round Roast and Steak
- Sirloin Tip Side
- Top Round Roast and Steak
- Bottom Round Roast and Steak
- Top Sirloin Steak
- Brisket, Flat Half

Of the ground beefs, ground sirloin is the leanest, followed by ground round and finally ground chuck.

Remember that grass-fed, grass-finished beef that is free of antibiotics is the healthiest choice! Grass-finished beef means that the cow was 100% grass fed and not fed grain the last 6 months to fatten it up.

For lean beef dining out recommendations, see the following chapter.

WEIRD FOOD COMBOS—MAKE UP YOUR OWN RULES!

When it comes to food combining, the sky is the limit. Plenty of healthy foods go together and since it is best to eat protein, carbohydrate and fat together, it is good for you to be creative and try new foods and new combos. Here are a few delicious, healthy combinations that I never thought sounded good, but when I actually got around to trying them, I realized how wrong I'd been:

- Eggs and sauerkraut
- Avocado, maple syrup and flax seeds
- Cottage cheese with coconut butter and sunflower seeds
- Blueberries in a green salad

CHOOSING HEALTHY GROCERIES

1. I will choose to write a grocery list using the "beginning shopper" suggestions and sample list from this chapter.

2. I will choose to write a grocery list using the guidelines provided in this chapter and go to the grocery store once this week and once next week.

3. I will choose to write a grocery list using the guidelines provided in this chapter and go to the grocery store once a week for a minimum of one month. I will also check the food labels on the foods I buy and make sure that I am buying foods with healthy, not damaged, fats, no added sugar, and high quality ingredients.

Chapter 10

Dining Out

Eating out can be a convenient as well as social dietary experience. In the best-case scenario, your dining out experience will be fun and nutritious. At worst, dining out is like walking through a culinary minefield. Many of my clients have expressed discomfort and even extreme anxiety when faced with social dining because they do not feel they are in control of what foods will be available to them; how the foods will be prepared; and how both of those factors will affect their health and waistline. In all honesty, I can completely relate! I am fortunate enough to live in an area where nutritious foods are more the norm than the exception, but my travels remind me that this option is not as prominent in other parts of the country or the world. I would like to present to you a dining out checklist that will help you to make the best food selections for any given situation.

WHEN DINING OUT, REMEMBER TO E.A.T.:

1. Eat a healthy appetizer before your meal instead of filling up on bread while you wait for your dinner. A salad, shrimp cocktail or chicken satay are several examples.

2. Ask questions--let your waitperson know what you want and ask for healthy recommendations.

3. Take your leftovers home--make it a point not to finish what is put in front of you. Most restaurants give you much more food than is wise to eat in one sitting.

If you follow these three suggestions, your dining out experience can be less stressful and a lot healthier. Below are some additional dining out tips that have been very successful for those of you who have a tendency to overeat. Remember that when you are eating the right foods for your body in the right amounts, you will not feel like overeating! When you eat the wrong foods for your body in the wrong ratios, you will have cravings and be inclined to overeat because your body isn't satisfied.

HELP WITH PORTIONS

1. Ask the waitperson to bring you a to-go container when they bring the food out to you. Eyeball what a healthy portion is and then immediately box up the excess: Out of sight, out of mind. Now you can just focus on the healthy portion that is is on your plate.

2. If you are familiar with the restaurant and the amount of food they serve, ask the waitperson at the time of ordering to box up the desired amount before serving you. That way when they do serve you, the portion will be more reasonable and your risk of overeating is lessened.

3. Push excess food off to the side of your plate when it first comes to you. Eyeball what is a reasonable portion and either make a mental note (not as safe) or physically mark (safer) what food you will eat versus what you will take with you. This option requires more willpower because the food will be on your plate as opposed to being boxed up and less conveniently accessible for cheating and having several extra bites. You can also ask the waitperson to bring an extra (smaller) plate so that you can put a serving from your entrée on it. Either of these options make it much easier to overeat since the food is right there in front of you and other people are overeating. Even the best of us can fall into the trap of eating less responsibly in this scenario. However, if you really don't see yourself following the above suggestions, try this option first. If it works--great! And if

not, try my other suggestions.

4. Make sure you know the ingredients of the food you are ordering. This is especially important if you have a food allergy or sensitivity. Sauces are commonly laced with gluten, egg, tomato, nuts, and citrus—all of which are common allergens. If your waitperson cannot tell you exactly what is in a sauce, it is best to enjoy your meal sans sauce and a side of olive oil instead.

SPEAK UP OR STAY HOME

One more thing I'd like to add to this section is that if you feel uncomfortable asking for what you want in a restaurant environment, you should limit your dining out frequency or choose places that already prepare foods in a healthy way. If you don't, then every time you dine out will be a step back on your road to improved health.

There is no shame in ordering food in a way that meets your health standards. Restaurants would be out of business if it weren't for your patronage. They provide a service and you pay for it. You should get what you want, so don't be shy to express what it is you need to make your experience enjoyable and stress-free. If the staff isn't respectful or if they do not willingly oblige reasonable requests, find a new restaurant or inform the management of your experience (if you don't want a confrontation, you can send an anonymous letter or phone in your complaint). You are not alone on this journey of trying every day to do your best to make healthy food choices and you shouldn't be deprived of having a fun night out that fits your health goals.

HEALTHY ORDERING GUIDE

Beverages

- Ice water or club soda (add lime, lemon, or orange for flavor)
- Coffee or tea without sugar. Stevia is a great non-calorie, non-

chemical sweetener. Real cream is preferable to powdered creamer.

- A maximum of one alcoholic beverage

Appetizers

- Broth-based soups
- Steamed or broiled vegetables
- Spring rolls in rice paper (not fried) or in lettuce/cabbage leaves
- Shrimp cocktail
- Chicken satay

Salads

- Ask for dressing on the side OR (since so many dressings use poor quality oils and added sweeteners) opt for olive oil and vinegar or lemon.

- If you are the type of person who does well with fat and protein, add meat, bacon and/or avocado. If you don't do as well with protein and fat, stick to a simple green salad.

- Use vinegar and lemon juice as a dressing. *Some people require more fat than others and need oil rather than vinegar or lemon juice.

Sandwiches

- Ask for spreads on the side so you can add the desired amount.

- Use mustard, lettuce, tomatoes, and toasted bread to improve taste without adding calories.

- If you need extra protein, fill your sandwich with chicken, turkey, tuna or beef.

- Consider having an open-faced sandwich to reduce your carbs and portion.

- Try a vegetarian sandwich with a few slices of cheese and lots of veggies (sprouts, cucumber, tomato, lettuce, onions). *This type of sandwich is satisfying to some people yet leave others unsatisfied and hungry. Observe which category you fall into.

- Ask for whole grain bread instead of white bread or rolls (rolls are higher in calories and starch since they are usually larger or more dense than sliced bread).

Entrees

- When it comes to the method of cooking for meat, ask for broiled, roasted or baked meats such as seafood, chicken, turkey, veal, London broil or beef tenderloin. If you require more fatty cuts, try ribeye or skirt steak.

- Cooking poultry without the skin drastically cuts calories and fat, so this can be great for some people or a disaster for others. If you require less fat, go skinless with poultry (either ask for the skin be removed prior to cooking or move it off to the side once it is served to you).

- Strip steak (Kansas or New York), filet mignon/tenderloin steak, T-bone, top sirloin/sirloin steak are all lean choices with less than 10 grams of total fat per serving/per 100 grams.

- Ask that the food be cooked without butter or oil and then add your own if appropriate for your metabolic type®.

- Only order a pasta dish if your body does really well with carbs and you can get a whole grain pasta.

- Marinara sauces and vegetarian red sauces tend to be lower in fat than cream-based sauces, so choose what works best for you.

Desserts

- Choose fresh fruit with or without cream

- Naturally sweet tasting tea (chocolate, caramel, vanilla or chai)

- Wait until you get home and have a small amount of dark chocolate or other low calorie, low sugar dessert.

FAT "BUZZ" WORDS

Pay special attention to descriptions on restaurant menus. There are key words that indicate whether the dish is high in fat and calories.

Choose what is ideal for your body type. Remember that some people need to eat more fat in order to lose body fat.

High-fat Indicators

- Alfredo
- Au gratin
- Batter dipped
- Béarnaise
- Béchamel
- Escalloped
- Beurre Blanc
- Breaded
- Creamy –
- Crispy
- Flaky
- Fried
- Hollandaise
- Parmagiana
- Puffed
- Tempura

Low-fat Indicators:

- Baked
- Broiled
- Flame cooked
- Grilled
- Steamed
- Smoked
- En croute
- Roasted
- Poached
- Marinara

BEWARE OF THE BUFFET

Buffets are a nightmare when it comes to trying to maintain healthful eating. The whole point of buffets for most people is to eat a lot of different foods and to go back many times to "get your money's worth." If you consider the amount of time and money you will put into trying to lose weight and be healthy, buffets are a complete rip-off. Saving five dollars on a buffet is not worth the hours you'll spend exercising, not to mention the emotional expense of feeling out of control with your eating and trying to work those excess calories off. Be preventative!

If you absolutely must attend a buffet meal, the best advice I can give is damage control by proper planning. Make a goal and a decision beforehand to:

1. Use a smaller plate.

2. Go up only once if you are not eating salad and pick the healthiest options available of the foods you like. DO NOT heap the plate full of food.

3. If you are eating salad, eat it first and keep it simple (don't pile

on every ingredient available). Choose several toppings such as sprouts, cucumbers, peppers, and either beans or olives and then top with vinaigrette. After you eat your salad, follow the guidelines for step number two.

4. Eat slowly and savor your food. Remember, this is not an opportunity to throw out all the good tools you have learned and make up for it later. Better health comes with daily health-conscious choices, not an I'll-make-better-choices-tomorrow attitude.

5. Don't eat everything on your plate. Walk away from those last few bites knowing you are sufficiently full and don't need the extra remaining calories.

CHOOSING HEALTHY DINING OUT EXPERIENCES

1. The next time I dine out, I will order all dressings and sauces on the side and I will add it myself a teaspoon at a time.

2. The next time I dine out, I will order all dressings/sauces on the side and I will stop eating when I am a 6-7 on the fullness scale (10 being overly full).

3. The next time I eat out, I will skip the bread basket and have a salad instead if I am really hungry; and/or, I will take half my dinner home in a to-go container for lunch the next day.

Section 3 – Fitness Made Simple

Chapter 11

Strength Training

As mentioned in Chapter 4, strength training is a critical component of total health and overall fitness. We all need to strength train at least once per week and many of us don't do even this. In a nutshell, strength training is a method of overloading your muscle tissue so that it breaks down and puts itself back together again even stronger than it was before.

TYPES OF STRENGTH TRAINING

There are several ways to strength train: free weights, weight stack machines, hydraulic machines, whole body vibration, calisthenics (such as pushups, pull-ups, lunges and squats using your own body weight for resistance), cables, resistance bands, tubing, medicine balls, and kettlebells, to name a few. It is good to have a variety to choose from because we all like different things. Variety allows us to stay interested so we stick with it for the long haul.

GET STRAIGHT, THEN STRENGTHEN

Before you start to strength train, it is critical to get a postural analysis by a skilled professional (Egoscue® therapist, physical therapist, or a personal trainer or yoga instructor with special training in postural therapy). Most people have postural dysfunctions (misaligned joints, asymmetries, feet that don't point forward, etc.) that over time will almost certainly lead to injuries, chronic pain, uneven wear on joints (which may require joint replacement surgery), muscle tightness and weakness. It is hazardous to your health to strengthen your body in a misaligned state. Reinforcing the postural dysfunction makes it that much harder to correct later on.

POSTURAL IMPROVEMENT ONE DAY AT A TIME

I strongly recommend a regular (daily if possibly) postural alignment regimen. I am not asking the impossible of you: It is completely within your means to start working on better posture immediately—and it feels great! I am not a morning person, but when I started waking up thirty minutes early to do my postural therapy exercises, it made a huge difference on how I felt the whole rest of the day. Sure, I was cranky about having to wake up earlier at first, but I have seen and felt great results and couldn't imagine myself not doing it. For more information, please visit www.egoscue.com. I also strongly recommend that you buy the book Pain Free by Pete Egoscue and Roger Gittines (it is inexpensive and has plenty of photos to make learning very easy).

You can also go to a yoga or Pilates class. The instructors are usually very knowledgeable and can teach you awareness so that you can preserve your body's natural alignment. Then you can fortify your body with strength training to reinforce proper alignment.

STRENGTH TRAINING BENEFITS

There are many benefits to strength training and this list is by no means exhaustive:

- Feeling and Looking Better–Strength training leads to increased lean muscle tissue, allowing you to look and feel more toned. Your stronger toned body is more capable of movement, which improves self-esteem and confidence.

- Increased Muscle Strength, Power, and Endurance–All of these benefits translates directly into having more freedom to do the active things you enjoy more often, for a longer period of time, and continue them later into life.

- Increased Metabolic Rate–Strength training increases the body's metabolic rate, causing the body to burn more calories throughout the day.

- Increasing and Restoring Bone Density–Inactivity and aging can lead to a decrease in bone density and brittleness. Studies have clearly proven that consistent strength training can increase bone density and prevent osteoporosis. Even starting a strength training program later in life has benefits for strengthening your bones and muscles.

- Injury Prevention–Strengthening muscles and joints helps prevent a wide variety of sports-related or life-related injuries.

- Improved Balance, Flexibility, Mobility and Stability–Stronger muscles that are properly trained to stabilize improves our balance, movement, and range of motion, which means more comfortable living and fewer falls or accidents.

- Aids Rehabilitation and Recovery–One of the best ways to heal many types of injuries is to strengthen muscles surrounding the injured area. The stronger your muscles, the quicker the healing process.

- Enhanced Performance in Sports or Exercise–No matter what your favorite sport or physical activity, with the proper strength training program, your performance can be dramatically improved.

- Aging Gracefully–There is no more important reason to making strength training a consistent part of your life, than to ensure you age gracefully. Physical activity keeps us alive and vibrant. Strength training ensures we are strong enough to participate in aerobic activities, outdoor recreation, and sports.

Strong seniors fall down less often. If they do fall down, their stronger bodies are more resilient, are injured less by the fall, and are able to heal more quickly after an injury.

- Improved Posture–A properly designed strength training program can help to balance out musculature by strengthening weak muscles that were previously incapable of supporting proper body alignment.

GETTING STARTED FOR BEGINNERS

Congratulations on your fitness endeavor! Feeling stronger and more fit is merely weeks away. First things first: you need a goal. We talked a lot about this at the beginning of the book. In case you don't remember, it is important to make sure your goals are S-M-A-R-T:

S-pecific
M-easurable,
A-ttainable,
R-elevant,
T-ime bound.

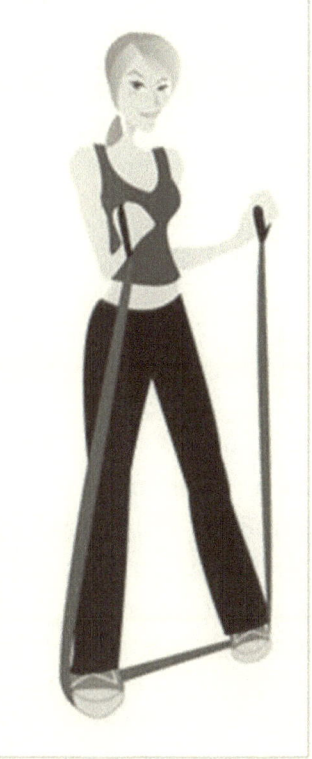

To give you an example, a reasonable strength training goal for a beginner is 1-3 workouts per week for 4 weeks with at least one exercise per major muscle group at 8-20 repetitions, 1-3 sets per exercise (I'll explain the wide variance in repetitions and sets in a moment). Notice that this goal is specific. I could get even more specific by listing the exact exercises:

Legs=Squats with dumbbells, Calf raises

Back=Seated row machine, Plank on elbows

Chest=Pushups

Arms=Biceps curls with dumbbells, Tricep dips on the floor

Abdominals=Crunches with feet on the wall, Side-to-side bends standing against a wall

This goal meets all the criteria of a SMART goal. If you completed this workout, you would know when you were finished (measurable), it is reasonable for a beginner (attainable), the exercises coincide with strengthening the whole body (relevant), and it is time bound (in four weeks, you can reassess).

CHOOSING SETS AND REPS

How many sets and repetitions you should complete depends on what you want to accomplish. If you are wanting to build some mass and a lot of strength, lower reps of 8-12, more sets (3+) and higher weight (a weight that fatigues your muscles in 8-12 reps) is recommended. If you want to primarily strengthen and tone without building much muscle mass, 12-15 reps and 1-2 sets is recommended. For those of you with goals to improve muscular endurance and tone, higher reps like 15-20 and 2-3 sets is preferred. If you are new to strength training, you need to start out with 1 set only of 12-15 reps per major muscle group. There is a lot of nervous system adaptation that takes place when you start a strength training program, so you need to allow 3-4 weeks for your body to make neural adaptations before you start adding sets.

CHOOSING PROPER WEIGHT

I mentioned in the previous section to select a weight that fatigues your muscles within the repetition range you select. If you choose a weight that is too easy, you won't get adequate results because your body doesn't have to work very hard to complete the set(s). Likewise, choosing a weight that is too heavy isn't good either since it increases your risk of injury (especially if you are a beginner).

If you are new to strength training, I urge you to start at the higher end of the repetition range (15-20 reps) and then select a weight that challenges you to fatigue by the last repetition. For example, if you are trying to build muscle and working within an 8-12 repetition range, start with a weight that fatigues you by 12 repetitions. After 4-6 weeks when both your muscles and joints are stronger, you can increase the weight and aim to fatigue your muscles in fewer repetitions.

The proper weight with which to train is discovered through trial and error. Make your best guess as to how much weight you can lift for the desired amount of reps. If you select a weight that you can only complete some of the reps, drop the weight. It is very important, especially for beginners, to gradually load your body. If you try to do too much too quickly, you greatly increase your chances of getting injured and then you won't be able to weight lift at all until you are healed! So I say again with caution: be safe and start slowly. Likewise, if you select a weight and are not fatigued after the set, choose a slightly higher weight.

There is a fine balance between choosing the right weight, a weight heavy enough to stimulate results, and a weight that is too light and easy. It will not take you long to find the right weight. After your first complete workout, you will know what is too heavy or too light. Write down the weight that you felt was best in terms of fatiguing you by the last repetition (12th, 15th, or 20th rep) for each exercise and this will be your starting out weight.

TIPS FOR MORE ADVANCED STRENGTH TRAINERS

If you are no stranger to strength training, this section is for you.

Here are some important questions to ask yourself:

Are you getting the results you want?

If you are getting the results you want, then you must be doing something right! Continue your current routine schedule and change the exercises, order of exercises, tempo or sets every 4-8 weeks to ensure continued adaptation and progress. After doing the same routine for longer than this, your body gets more and more efficient at it and you work less hard and therefore your progress starts to plateau.

Are you happy with your current program?

It is important to change your routine so that you don't get bored or burned out. As mentioned above, this should be done every 4-8 weeks. The saying "No pain, no gain" is not good advice. Your routine should not hurt you; it should challenge you. You should have a strength training routine that you enjoy, not because it is easy, but because it is well-suited to both your strengths and weaknesses.

Working with a personal trainer and having a program designed especially for you is a great way to ensure that you have a workout regimen that will keep you challenged and well balanced.

How often do you change your routine?

In case you missed it the first two times: every 4-8 weeks! This time-line applies even if you really like your current program. It won't benefit you nearly as much to do the same routine for months on end. Change and new challenges are important. You can return to your old routine again after you have tried something else in between.

MIX IT UP!

Here are some suggestions for mixing things up and giving you some variety and challenge:

- **Jump Intervals**–Try a 1-2 minute jump roping interval between sets and/or exercises. This will increase your caloric burn and is a great endurance conditioning tool.

- **Wild Card Workout**–Do a different routine one day per week or try a new exercise on a certain day (e.g., every Fri).

- **Have a Ball**–try some traditional exercises on an exercise ball. For example, for exercising your chest, lay your shoulders and head on a ball instead of lying on a bench. The extra stability work by your glutes, low back and obliques is a nice challenge.

- **Add a Day of Yoga**–Yoga is terrific for helping you keep your muscles balanced and helping to prevent injuries.

- **Cardio Intervals**–After working a body part (e.g., legs), do a 55-minute cardio interval.

- **Face Your Fears**–Don't avoid exercises that are harder for you! This is a common mistake and one that ensures muscular imbalance. Find a way that does not cause you pain (a little muscle soreness doesn't count) to strengthen an area that you have been avoiding because it is harder. Too often people do exercises that are easy for them, usually because they are already strong in the area that the exercise is focusing. Challenge yourself!

CHOOSING STRENGTH

1. I choose to start strengthening my body by: a) Meeting with a qualified personal trainer and getting an individualized routine, b) Going to a yoga class once per week so an instructor can supervise my posture, and/or c) Doing one at-home strength training workout per week

2. I choose to strengthen my body twice per week consistently either at a gym or at home using the guidelines from this chapter.

3. I choose to strengthen my body by integrating the exercise ball, jump rope, cardio intervals and/or yoga for each of my three strength training sessions per week for a minimum of one month.

Chapter 12

Cardiovascular Health

R egular aerobic exercise is a fundamental necessity to overall health. It has been found to lower blood pressure, improve HDL cholesterol, improve body composition (lose fat), increase lung capacity, condition heart muscle so it pumps more blood with less strain, increase stamina and endurance, improve mood--the list goes on and on. With so many benefits, you can't afford not to make aerobic exercise a part of your life. It doesn't matter how in shape you are right now; the important thing is to start moving! Here are some steps that will make getting started easier:

1. Pick a form of exercise that you like (e.g., dancing, walking, biking, trampoline, swimming, etc.).

2. Start with a manageable goal of frequency and duration. For example, three times per week for ten minutes. As you adapt to this original goal and feel that you can do more, you can gradually increase how often and how long you exercise.

3. Have a longer-term goal to work toward. This can be anything from being able to do a specific hike that you weren't able to do before, to running in a marathon. Make your goal something that you will feel proud of once you've accomplished it.

4. Enjoy your success and have follow up goals. Continually revise your goals so you don't get bored and give up. Nothing feels as low as reaching your first long-term goal and having nothing afterward to look forward to. If you acknowledge this up front,

you will save yourself the heartache. I've seen too many clients reach their long-term weight loss goal and only have fleeting joy. How ironic is that—after spending months or even years working toward a goal and then only enjoying it for ten minutes?! You owe yourself more than that, so I'm telling you now that you should celebrate your accomplishment and have other irons in the fire to look forward to and keep you motivated.

GETTING THE MOST OUT OF YOUR WORKOUT

Exercise has so many benefits, but let's face it, we all get bored sometimes. This section gives you some tips to try along your journey to help keep you motivated!

Increase the calorie burn and make your cardio workout more fun with these intensity-boosting ideas (Raskin, 2006).

- **Push it with your playlist**—Speed up whenever the chorus of a song is played.

- **TV training**—Kick up your intensity during commercials. If you're watching a news channel, sprint for 30 seconds every time you hear the president's name and/or when a different news reporter starts talking.

- **Drop and give yourself 10**—When you are doing cardio, either outside or on a machine, stop every five minutes and do five push ups and five crunches.

- **Go car spotting**—Running or walking outside? When a red car passes you, sprint for 10 seconds; a black car, 20 seconds; and a white one, 30 seconds. Or make up your own system based on the models or colors of cars. (Idea taken from Jennifer Nicole Lee, creator of the DVD series Fabulously Fit Moms.)

- **Add 10 minutes in the morning**—No matter what your normal workout schedule is, waking up 10 minutes earlier in the morning and taking a walk around the block (or, alternatively, simply dancing to your morning radio show for 10 minutes) will let you start off your day with a faster-burning metabolism and, most likely, head off to work in a better mood than usual. *Calorie-burning boost: 275 calories per week*

- **Work out with a faster partner**—Whether it's in the gym or on the neighborhood track, a fit buddy will challenge you to keep up and exercise at a higher intensity. It's the friendliest way to kick your own butt! Plus, workouts go faster accompanied by good conversation. *Calorie-burning boost: Simply increasing your walk from 3 mph to 4 mph will burn almost 100 extra calories in 60 minutes.*

INTERVAL TRAINING

When you alternate high-intensity cardio work with moderate-intensity recovery periods, you boost your calorie burning and increase your fitness level. This will help you break through plateaus.

Several of the above-mentioned examples demonstrate fun ways to mix interval training into your cardio regimen. Here are the general guidelines so you can experiment:

1. Warm up for 5 minutes.

2. Increase your speed or resistance on the machine (or outside) for 2-5 minutes.

3. Return to your usual pace for 5 minutes.

4. Next, continue with short bursts interspersed with a moderate pace for the rest of your workout.

5. Cool down for 5 minutes at a slower pace.

6. When you're ready to progress, make the intense part of the interval longer and decrease the recovery time (but never to less than 30 seconds). For example, you could do 6 minutes at a higher speed (instead of 5) and recover for 3 minutes (instead of 5).

Interval training not only makes your workouts more interesting, but can make a big difference in your strength, endurance and calorie burn!

CALCULATE YOUR TARGET HEART RATE

Depending on your fitness goal, it is helpful to calculate a heart rate range to suit your goal. As a general guideline, the following percentages can be used to calculate an appropriate exercise intensity for different fitness levels:

Beginner or low fitness level...50% - 60%
Average fitness level...........60% - 70%
High fitness level...............75% - 85%

Choose which percentage range matches your goals and then plug it into the formula below (The Karvoven Formula). Your resting heart rate is your heart rate when you aren't exercising.

- For the most accurate results, take your pulse at your neck (carotid pulse) or your wrist (radial pulse). Don't use your thumb since it has its own pulse!

- Count your heart beats, starting with zero, for one minute. This is your resting heart rate. For more accuracy, you can follow these instructions and calculate your resting heart rate for three mornings and then take the average.

Karvoven Formula

220 - Age = Maximum Heart Rate
Max Heart Rate - Resting Heart Rate x Intensity + Resting Heart Rate
= Training Heart Rate

Knowing your target heart rate will help keep you motivated throughout your workout since it gives you something for which to aim. Working out within this range will also help you achieve your goals faster.

TRACKING YOUR PROGRESS

It can be motivating to write down your daily exercise accomplishments. Here is an example but feel free to make up your own:

Date	Time	Distance	Other

CHOOSING CARDIOVASCULAR HEALTH

1. I choose to select a type of aerobic exercise that I enjoy and do 10 minutes of it (less, if I am physically unable) twice this week.

2. I choose to do aerobic exercise for 20 minutes or more three times this week in my target heart rate zone.

3. I choose to do aerobic exercise for 30 minutes or more 3-7 times this week in my target heart rate zone. I will accomplish this goal by choosing a combination of types of aerobic exercise such as fast walking, swimming, dancing, biking, or taking an aerobics class at the gym or using a cardio machine such as an elliptical trainer.

Chapter 13

Flexibility & Posture

S tretching is a very controversial topic lately, but it didn't used to be. Stretching before and after a workout was something that was accepted as part of the workout itself. In my experience, people who stretch enjoy it and comment on how good they feel afterward. I have never had a client who finished stretching and said that they didn't feel better than before they had stretched. Recently though, stretching has been questioned for validity, safety and even blamed for increasing a person's risk of injury.

According to UC Berkeley's Wellness Letter (2007) and many other fitness books, "stretching improves flexibility" and "flexibility is a key element of fitness." However, other credible sources have found that stretching may not have the benefits we once believed it to have. An example is a large Australian study which concluded that stretching prior to working out did not significantly reduce one's risk of leg injury (Pope, et al., 2000.) The jury is out and may always be out on whether stretching has credible scientific data to support its benefit(s). As for its risk of increasing your chances of an injury, there is not enough data to support this. One thing that we do know is that it sure feels great to stretch!

FLEXIBILITY IN HISTORY

Many age-old fitness traditions pivot around (or at least include) stretching: yoga, Pilates, dance, Capoeira and most martial arts. If stretching offered no benefit, would it be such an integral component to so many health practices? I don't think so. Arguments about whether stretching decreases our chances of getting injured aside, there is a great deal of data to support how flexibility is intricately linked to posture and proper alignment.

DYNAMIC TENSION

When a muscle or an entire muscle group is too tight, it pulls the body in its direction. When a muscle is too flexible, it may not be strong enough to keep you posturally balanced against the opposing muscle(s). This relationship of opposing muscle groups and how they work together to create balance in our bodies is called dynamic tension. We've all seen someone whose dynamic tension is severely dysfunctional: they are the person leaning so far forward that they look like they are going to fall over. Even if you aren't a health professional, you can look at someone with posture like that and know that something is very wrong.

Perhaps it is not stretching or flexibility we should be looking to for answers, but rather how our muscles work together (or against each other) to achieve balance or tensegrity. Put another way, "All structures in the universe are supported by a balance between tension and compression, between 'push' and 'pull,'" (retrieved from http://www.anatomytrains.com/explore/tensegrity/explained). Striving for this kind of muscular and postural balance is the key to a healthy body that craves movement rather than shying away from it.

GRAVITY: FRIEND AND FOE

Unless you are an astronaut, gravity affects your body every second of every day. This is information you can use to your advantage or, if ignored, can lead to very undesirable and dysfunctional posture over time. As a child, I was always extremely active, especially with dance. While I was kinesthetically aware, I would discover many years later that my postural awareness was very limited. Many of you may think, as I did well into adulthood, that posture is about standing or sitting up tall and not slouching. It wasn't until reading Pain Free by Pete

172

Egoscue and Roger Gittines that my concept of posture was forever changed (I highly recommend this book. It is full of easy to read information about your body's ideal posture, common dysfunctions, and most importantly, how to return to a functional, healthy body. There are pictures and clear descriptions making it incredibly user-friendly.

Another excellent resource is Anatomy Trains by Thomas Myers). I was shocked that there were postural dysfunctions in my very own body that I had never noticed! It was like putting on a pair of colored glasses (except the glasses I had put on made my left shoulder higher than my right, my head ever so slightly tilted to the left, and my right shoulder rotate forward!). I was horribly depressed for about five minutes until I realized what a gift I had been given: now that I was aware of what was wrong, I could change it and the tools were right in front of me.

There are exercises and poses that use gravity to reposition our muscles and joints in a pain-free and somewhat passive way. I now do an hour of what author Pete Egoscue calls "e-cises" first thing every morning. Little by little, changes are happening. I am observing an improvement in my alignment and with those changes, I am losing those little aches and pains that so many of us put up with because we didn't think we had a choice. There is another choice and it is spending anywhere from twenty minutes to an hour of "being in your body," working with your alignment and helping your body come back to its designed posture.

WAYS YOU CAN IMPROVE YOUR POSTURE

Take Yoga

It isn't just for people who are super flexible, even though this is the common misconception. My husband calls yoga "pretzel" and I know that he is not alone in believing that people who do yoga bend into positions that would put a circus contortionist to shame. Sure, yogis can do amazing things with their bodies. But do you really believe that they were just born doing stretches and hand-stands?

Through yoga and discipline, they have learned and perfected amazing strength and poise. Yoga is incredibly balancing to the body and the mind.

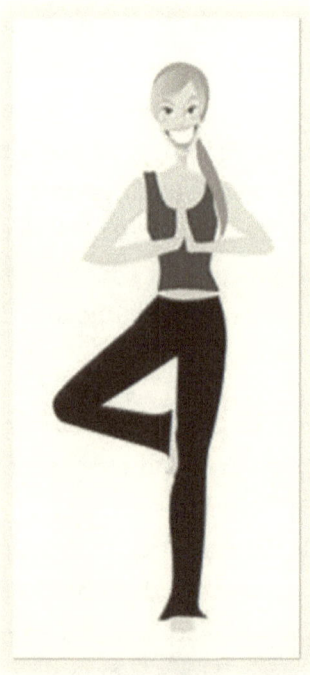

If you have never done it and are intimidated, take a very beginner class at your gym or local yoga studio. You can also buy a tape or DVD that you can follow in the privacy of your own home (just make sure you have enough room!). Some yoga instructors provide private instruction so that you can get one-on-one yoga help. If you are a busy, impatient or an on-the-go-most-of-the-time kind of person, you will either love or hate yoga right away. If you hate it right away and find it painfully slow and boring, you need it more than anyone. Don't quit after your first class. Make yourself go for a month (at least once per week) and I guarantee that you will develop a deeper appreciation for your own body and for yoga.

Stretch at Home

Dedicate even ten minutes per day to keeping your body limber. Emphasize stretches in areas where you are especially tight. You can get ideas from classes, exercise videos, the fitness channel, or from a fitness professional. For your convenience, I have included some illustrations.

Use A Foam Roller

These are brilliant in their simplicity! They are firm cylinders of foam that you roll your body against. Repetitive use of a foam roller loosens you up, is great for myofascia release (fibrous netting that encases our muscles), and hurts so good! Regular rolling improves posture, range of motion and reduces tight-ness.

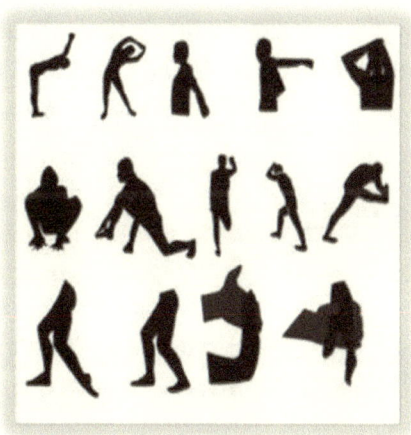

Get Rolfed

Rolfing is one of the best ways to realign and break up fascial tightness in your body. Rolfing is a form of bodywork that works to structurally realign the body over the course of a series of sessions. It is intense and even painful at times, but this form of bodywork will definitely allow your body to move more freely, stand up taller and feel more balanced overall.

See A Chiropractor or Physical Therapist

A good chiropractor will not only help you identify how your body is misaligned, but will combine their adjustment with teaching about daily exercises you can do so your body can learn to hold itself in alignment. A good physical therapist can help make manual adjustments to your body as well, and they are all about giving you homework: daily exercises or stretches that you can do to allow your body to heal and prevent future injuries through improved alignment and strength.

Go to an Egoscue® Clinic

As I have already attested to, I think Egoscue® should be tried by everyone for at least two weeks. Once you feel how positively your body responds to improved alignment, flexibility and "communication" as a unified whole, you will be forever grateful. Go to www.egoscue.com to locate a clinic near you. They will take posture photos so that you can track your progress over time.

Do Egoscue® at Home

If you aren't near a clinic or for some reason just don't want to go, there are many books with clear pictures and descriptions that can help you to do Egoscue® daily in the privacy of your own home.

Their website also has some "menus," lists of exercises and stretches plus photos, to help you start right away. You can even do your own "before" posture photos so that you can track your postural improvements over time.

CHOOSING HEALTHY POSTURE

1. I choose to spend a minimum of five minutes one day this week stretching.

2. I choose to spend a minimum of five minutes three times this week stretching. I will strongly consider taking a beginner yoga class and having a professional assess my posture.

3. I will get a copy of Pain Free from the library (or buy a copy). Then I will look at the three posture conditions, assessing which condition I come closest to. I will then go through the "pain free" exercises recommended for that condition four times in a week.

Chapter 14

Rest

O f all the things we've learned about the world, science, and our bodies, it is still not completely understood why we need sleep and why we die if deprived of it for too long. What we do know is that sleep is an essential part of life and without enough, we break down mentally, emotionally and physically. Sleep is important for allowing the repair systems of the body to take place uninterrupted, our thoughts to organize and store memories, and even a time for us to sort out our emotions.

But rest is another important health factor, separate from sleep, that we require to replenish ourselves. Conscious downtime where our minds are free to drift and explore, our physical body able to breathe deeply and feel whatever it feels, is a need that we mistake for luxury instead of scheduling it as a priority. Even five minutes a day of uninterrupted rest time has physical, emotional, and mental benefits.

We push ourselves in so many arenas in life that we forget that rest (relaxation) is a vital component to our overall health and success.

Adequate rest improves mental, physical, and emotional strength.

Without enough rest, we will lose interest in things that were once important to us and our successes for which we worked so hard will fade away. Our minds and bodies will force us to slow down, because without rest, we cannot healthily move forward.

OVERTRAINING

From an exercise and recovery perspective, even though it seems counterintuitive, rest is important for progress. Our bodies get stronger during the rest periods following exercise rather than during the exercise itself. Without rest, we burn out and show signs of overtraining.

SIGNS OF OVERTRAINING

- Elevated resting heart rate (5-10 beats above normal)
- Fatigue
- Irritability
- Poor sleep
- Poor appetite
- Depression
- Increased susceptibility to colds
- Increased injuries
- Lack of motivation
- Sore joints and muscles
- Headaches
- Drop in sport/exercise performance

For general recovery and muscle tissue repair following strength training one should observe a 48-hour period of rest for the major muscle groups (excluding calves and abdominals). For cardiovascular exercise, 1-2 days of more gentle aerobic exercise is recommended to prevent overtraining. These are general guidelines and you may find that you require more recovery time. Listen to your body and remember that sometimes less is more.

PAMPER YOURSELF

Taking special care of yourself is always appreciated. Don't make it an annual occurrence—you deserve more frequent special treatment! It doesn't have to be expensive or even time consuming, but it does require you to get into the proper mindset that you are taking some time out of your busy schedule to do something restorative for yourself. Here are some great ways of pampering yourself either on an exercise day or a non-exercise day:

- Rub arnica on sore muscles

- Use essential oils (e.g., lavender) in your bath or lotions to soothe tired muscles

- Take a bath with Epsom salts

- Get a massage

- Take a hot tub

- Put on some of your favorite music, close your eyes and breathe

- Give yourself a facial, manicure or pedicure (men too!)

- Make yourself your favorite healthy meal and eat by candlelight

- Give yourself a beach day (or whatever source of nature is within proximity)

- Go on a leisurely stroll and picnic

- Allow yourself to take a nap

- Do gentle stretching

- Meditate

- Do something creative that you enjoy (drawing, writing, painting, etc.)

By treating yourself well and allowing your body and mind to rejuvenate, you will not only look and feel more refreshed, but you will get more accomplished in your lifetime and feel more successful. Think of it as charging your batteries so that you can go about life with renewed vigor!

BREATHING

We breathe approximately 22,000 times per day. You can make an incredible difference to your mental, emotional and physical well- being if you learn to breathe properly. An amazing technique that I learned from Brian Bradley at Egoscue® is called East-West Breathing. The name east-west describes the direction that your waist goes when you breathe into your diaphragm as opposed to the chest or shoulders. When you see people breathe and their whole upper body rises and falls with each breath, this is called north-south breathing. North-south breathing is shallow. The lower portion of the lungs do not soak up air. In north-south breathing, the accessory muscles of the upper body (trapezius, levator scapula, pec minor, and scalenes) are recruited with every breath to move the shoulders up and down in an attempt to artificially create space for the lungs to take in more air. This isn't their job! Those muscles are intended to stabilize the head and shoulders as well as perform during movements such as lifting, pulling and pushing. Recruiting them to do a job that they weren't designed to do and asking them to do it 22,000 times every day is a disaster waiting to happen.

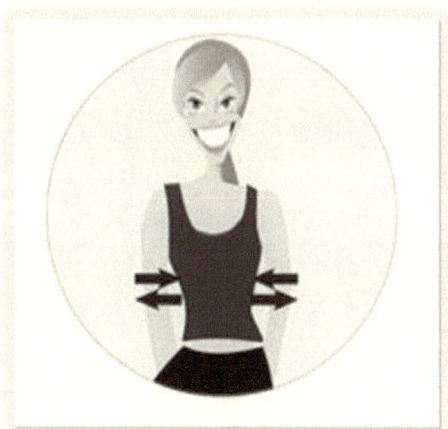

Learning to breathe east-west style takes some time and patience. The easiest position to feel if you are doing it correctly is laying on your back.

1. Lay on the floor on your back with your knees bent.

2. Place your fingers on the sides of your waist just below the ribcage.

3. Take a deep breath in and try to take the breath from your abdominal area. You should feel your waist push against your fingers. Don't be discouraged if you can't get it right away. Practice!

The pressure you will feel on either side of your waist when you are able to do it is a reflection of the intra-abdominal pressure created when the diaphragm moves downward to make room for your lungs to take in more air. This pressure is beneficial to your lower back as it plays a large role in spinal stability. Intra-abdominal pressure also strengthens your deep abdominal muscles. The increased movement of your diaphragm is great for digestion because it increases peristalsis (wavelike movement of the intestines to push food through).

For more information about east-west breathing, I recommend getting a copy of the DVD series East-West Breathing by the Egoscue Method®. Not only does it explain the benefits of this style of breathing in great detail but the last DVD includes exercises to improve your breathing and posture.

Movement classes such as martial arts, Qi gong and yoga as well as voice or wind instrument training also emphasize proper breathing. Try whichever option appeals to you and start right away. Make the most out of those breaths!

CHOOSING REST

1. I choose to spend five minutes this week doing absolutely nothing except breathing and appreciating being alive.

2. I choose to spend a minimum of five minutes 3-4 times this week relaxing and I will pamper myself once this week (see above list or create your own healthy pampering idea).

3. I choose to sleep 6-8 hours per night at least five nights a week for a minimum of one month and I will pamper myself weekly.

Section 4 – Maintenance: How to Make it Last

Chapter 15

Maintenance and Self-Monitoring: A Perfect Marriage

Reaching one's goals in some ways is much harder than maintaining them, but this is only true if you know that some level of constant accountability must remain. It is easier to slip off track if you do not monitor yourself. This is why I am dedicating a chapter to the art of self-monitoring and its benefits.

HOW DO I KNOW IF I AM MAINTAINING?

The only way to keep track of your healthy accomplishments is to have a system that allows you to monitor those accomplishments.

You'll need to know several things to determine if you are maintaining your results. First, you must know which aspects to track and have a place to record your findings. For example, for weight maintenance, several aspects you should track are your weight, body fat percentage, and body measurements.

RECORDING WEIGHT

For weighing yourself, you should use the same scale once per week at the same time of day and record the number in a journal/notebook or on a sheet of paper. I recommend having a notebook dedicated to monitoring your health maintenance. When you weigh yourself weekly, observe if the number fluctuates greatly or is the same every week. Several pounds of fluctuation are normal, so don't be alarmed. If your weight fluctuates by more than five pounds, it is worthwhile to look further into your behaviors to see if exercise or diet is varying a lot and affecting your weight each week

The tracking of behaviors ties directly into one of the other useful means of weight maintenance. You will need to know which behaviors affect what you are trying to track (in this case, weight maintenance). For example, does your weight stay the same if you exercise for thirty minutes five times per week? If you eat three large meals a day, does your weight go up? Asking yourself these questions and adapting your behaviors accordingly will allow you to avoid large changes in your weight/body fat. When you keep a weekly eye on these health factors, it is much easier to make small changes and maintain your weight rather than allowing a month of changes to happen before making any corrections.

WAYS OF KEEPING TRACK OF YOUR BODY-FAT AND SIZE

Aside from recording your weekly weight in your health journal, as I mentioned before, another good method for monitoring progress or maintenance is to have regular body fat tests. There are many different types of body fat tests.

- Hydrostatic or underwater weighing

- Bio-electrical impedance -hand-held -scale -ultrasound -electrode

- Skin Calipers

Hydrostatic or underwater weighing is the most accurate for estimating body fat percentage, but also inconvenient and time consuming—you need to find a facility that offers it and the test itself can take about an hour (from start to finish).

Other more convenient and fairly accurate types of body fat tests include bio-electrical impedance either with a handheld tester; step- on scale; higher-end testers where you need another person to administer the test (electrodes are placed at certain points on your body and you lay still while the tester presses the "calculate body fat" button); ultrasound body fat testers; and calipers (a.k.a. the "pinch" test). I encourage you to try different methods and choose one that is convenient for you to repeat monthly so you can record and keep track of increases or decreases in your muscle to fat ratio.

BODY MEASUREMENTS

Body measurements are also a good way of gauging weight maintenance. You can have a professional do full body measurements at a set interval (monthly, every three months, twice a year, etc.), or you can learn to do a waist circumference test yourself. I recommend both. It is good to have someone else measure arm, chest, waist, navel, hips, thigh, and calf, but you can also do a waist circumference test in front of the mirror (so you can see if you are lining up the measuring tape properly). Once per month is a reasonable frequency.

WAIST CIRCUMFERENCE TEST

The waist to hip ratio used to be the more popular standard for assessing health with a measuring tape. However, since it is an indicator of abdominal fat, the waist circumference is a useful (and one step easier than the waist to hip ratio) alternative that provides the necessary health screening info.

Use a flexible or cloth tape so that it lays flat on your skin and measure at the line of your navel (bellybutton). Do this on your bare skin. Record your measurement in your journal. Also record if you measured over clothes or not since they can add anywhere from ¼ -¾ of an inch.

Women are aiming for 35 inches or less. Men are aiming for 40 inches or less.

It is better to be shaped like a pear rather than an apple. The "apple" shape indicates excess belly fat. Those shaped like apples are at increased risk of heart disease, stroke, diabetes, and hypertension.

METHODS FOR KEEPING TRACK OF HEALTHY BEHAVIORS

Food journaling or some form of record keeping of your food/beverage intake is very helpful for long-term weight maintenance. It is all too easy to become so distracted by other aspects of our lives that we lose track of taking care of ourselves.

Getting Off Track

Unless you are keeping record of your day-to-day health behaviors, there are many ways to slip into habits that will lead you right back to where you started. Examples of this are:

- Getting busy at work and skipping lunch and then stopping somewhere on your way home from work to get a candy bar, fast food, sugary/caffeinated drinks, etc.

- Not planning out your meals and buying convenience foods that are overly processed and caloric instead OR filling up on convenience foods that aren't as nutritious. Both ruin your appetite for an actually nutritious meal.

- Not bothering to refill your water bottle throughout the day and instead drinking soda, coffee, or other processed drinks.

These examples are all too common and they happen when we stop paying attention—so don't fall victim to being oblivious! You can keep yourself on track by doing a food journal several times each week and reviewing it for red flag foods, drinks, portion sizes, and the above mentioned "pitfall" behaviors.

Food Portion Monitoring

If you are eating right for your metabolic type®, your body will automatically adjust to eating the right portions of food to satisfy your energy needs. If you are eating the wrong foods for your body or eating the wrong ratios of the right foods (i.e., too much carb, not enough fat or vice versa), you will struggle with your portions and controlling your weight. If you fall into the category of someone who needs to monitor their food portions, there are many options to fit the different lifestyle needs we have. Read the options here and pick which one(s) you think will work best for you.

Food Scales

Have you ever measured out your food before eating it? Food scales have become quite popular, but they aren't for everyone. Food scales can be digital, dials, or adjustable discs that allow you to see exactly how much food you are eating. Before turning up your nose at the idea, give it the old "I'll try anything once" approach. You can learn a lot by experimentally weighing your food for even just one day.

If you want precision and are not interested in guessing your portions, a food scale is a great option. You can weigh out the correct portion sizes when you cook, make your lunch, or pack snacks. As an added bonus, the more you use your food scale, the better you will become at intuitively eating correct portions. This is good since it isn't practical to take your food scale out to a restaurant or when you are traveling.

Measuring Cups

If food scales don't appeal to you, there is also the good old-fashioned measuring cup. Like the food scale, you can learn a lot by experimentally measuring your food for a day. Are you an accurate eye-baller or do you frequently underestimate a healthy portion? By using a measuring cup and measuring spoons, you will become quite good at eating and drinking more reasonable portions. Even so, if you do not use these measurement tools daily, I recommend revisiting them from time to time to make sure that you aren't getting rusty and overestimating food servings.

FOOD JOURNAL

Recording your daily food intake does wonders for accountability. Many times I have been told by clients that they did not eat something "bad for them" because they didn't want to write it down! Even if this is not the case, food journaling is great for you to see what your eating trends are with frequency, amount, and variety.

Food journaling--the detailed documentation of one's daily food and liquid intake--is just one more example of how our dreams become reality. Try keeping a food journal for two days during the week and one day on the weekend. Document everything you consume for those three days.

Types of Food Journals

Food journals have come a long way over the years. In the past, food journaling was limited to writing everything down in a notebook or on a piece of paper, but now we have more options. There is great

value in the old notebook method, but for those that are on/by a computer or cell phone all day, there are a variety of electronic options.

Electronic Food Journals

Many health and fitness websites have online food journal options (such as MyFitnessPal) that make it easy for you to document your dietary intake. If you spend a good part of the day by a computer, this is a great option since convenience is a key in establishing a new behavior.

Online Reminders

You can also send email reminders to yourself to journal (put it on your computer calendar and if your calendar has the option to send an email reminder, do it!). You can ask friends, family members, and health professionals such as a personal trainer or a nutritionist to email you reminders as well. If you work with a trainer or a nutritionist, email your food journal to them. Establish a schedule with them for the frequency that you will send them your journal (daily, weekly, biweekly, etc.). Some of my clients prefer food journaling spreadsheets which they can fill out and email back to me.

It is convenient and helps them stay accountable. Increasing your accountability will strengthen your attention to your diet and open the doors for support and healthy recommendations.

Smart Phones & Wearable Health Trackers

Smart phones are a very convenient method for tracking food intake and exercise output.

Find an app that you like and that will send you reminders (such as MyFitnessPal).

Another great option is to use a wearable health tracker around your wrist or finger to log food, track movement, and get reminders & encouragement throughout the day (examples include FitBit, Garmin, Oura Ring, Motiv Ring, Moov Now, and Misfit). Technology in this area continually improves and the options continue to grow.

Photo Food Journaling

For those of you who believe in the whole "a picture is worth a thousand words" concept, I've come up with the perfect food journal system for you: photo food journaling. You can use your cell phone camera or actually carry around a small digital camera with you and take a picture of everything you eat or drink prior to consumption. If you don't eat the whole portion, take a picture of what is left so you can see how much you ate. Photo food journaling is a great option if you just aren't interested in writing things down or if you have a hard time estimating portions. Most people underestimate how much they eat when they food journal any-way—sometimes by as much as 25%--so this method is great for accuracy. If you work with a trainer or nutritionist, you can email them the photos for added accountability.

Does Food Journaling Help with Weight Loss?

Self-monitoring works as one of the most effective tools for maintaining weight loss over time. Numerous clinical studies have compared weight loss groups in which one group food journals on a regular basis while the other group does not. Reviews of these studies show consistent agreement that persons who record at least 75% of their eating and exercising behaviors lost significantly more weight and maintained weight loss effectively over time compared to their non-self-monitoring counterparts (Kirschenbaum, 2000).

Self-monitoring allows you to reflect upon your behaviors and choices. For the best and most accurate results, I recommend that you record your food intake right away and not wait to record it (oh, how quickly we forget!).

FOOD GUIDANCE SYSTEMS

Not everything works for everyone. For those of you who are opposed to keeping a food journal, some of the following options may help. Food guidance systems such as the one provided by https://www.supertracker.usda.gov/default.aspx--the official dietary guidelines for Americans--can provide structure and accountability by supplying you with specific amounts of foods to eat within every food group, activity goals, and worksheets to record daily dietary intake. While the worksheet is similar to a food journal, it differs in that you merely write down the amount of food you had in each group (format provided) and tally it up over the course of the day, rather than starting from a blank piece of paper and writing down exactly what was eaten and when. For some of us, this small detail will make all the difference.

Food Checklists

For an option that is similar to the food guidance system, food checklists work well and are easier for some people. A food checklist is exactly what it sounds like: a piece of paper with food selections on it that you check off throughout the day once they have been eaten. You can use your metabolic typing® guidelines as the basis for the food groups and amounts to have on your checklist. Simply write down the different food categories and the amounts for each that you have determined works well for you and put checkboxes next to them. This method is great for a quick recording of one's daily intake. It doesn't provide as much detail as the other methods, but as long as it helps you be accountable and make better food choices, it is a credible food-tracking option.

MENU PLANS

If you need more structure than either food journaling or food guidance systems provide, you will do best if given daily menus for all of your snacks and meals. To ensure proper nutrient intake and variety as well as caloric balance, this is something that a licensed nutritionist or registered dietician should do. Go to www.mt-advisors.info/to locate a nutrition professional near you or call your doctor and ask for a referral. Most good insurances will cover nutrition appointments after your deductible is met.

EXERCISE JOURNAL

Exercise recording is another helpful form of self-monitoring. Write down your activity and how long you did it. It may also be useful to record the intensity/difficulty of the exercise and how you felt afterward. Tracking your activity from week to week allows you to see how regularly you are moving your body, what sorts of activity your body is getting, and how the length of your workouts may change over time.

Some of my clients have exercise journals from when they first started strength training and are thrilled when they look back and see the weight they started lifting compared to what they can lift now.

They are proud of the changes they have made in their bodies. They can also see how their aerobic endurance has changed by how long they can last when they are riding a bike or walking/running. It is these observations that keep motivation and self-esteem high; aside from the physical improvement to our health, that is what results are for!

MIND OVER MATTER

Affirmations are a big part of success in any area, especially health. I explained in detail in Chapter 2 how powerful our thoughts are in effecting our behavior. We are in control of our thoughts and our thoughts guide our actions. If you think to yourself at the beginning of each day that you care about your health and happiness and will therefore eat healthily, nourish your body with water, and schedule exercise into your day, you have a much stronger likelihood of accomplishing these goals than if you leave it all to chance.

Identify what is important to you, prioritize your health and do what it takes to make the necessary steps happen (go to the grocery store so that you have the supplies for eating a healthy breakfast, pack a healthy lunch and snacks, and make a healthy dinner). It won't happen magically and it won't happen just because you want it— thoughts are important but they must be combined with action. Daily affirmations and goals are an excellent first step. Follow through with taking action and you will accomplish your goals.

Avoiding Holiday Pitfalls

No longer are the holidays limited to the latter part of the year. Most of us have a "holiday" -- any celebration that includes food as the center of attention-- at least twice a month, year-round. This makes your job of healthy eating and avoiding food traps more challenging, unless of course, you have a plan. Rather than being caught off-guard and feeling controlled by food-focused situations, take control and develop a strategy. Holidays are for celebrating, not sabotaging your health goals. You can have fun without under- mining your efforts.

Holidays are often used as an excuse to indulge. While an occasional indulgence is fine, eating and drinking an excess of 17,500 to 35,000 calories (5-10lbs worth) is a pitfall best avoided. Holiday weight fluctuations are an unnecessary evil that are totally avoidable. Here are some suggestions to help you evade the physical and emotional stress of holiday weight yo-yo-ing:

- Most importantly, accept the fact that it is your responsibility to change and commit to behaving differently.

- Map out your hidden holidays. Mark your calendar with all the food-heavy events you expect to encounter in the months ahead, not just the big ones. For example, include birthday parties (work, family, and friends), baby or bridal showers, Fourth of July barbecues, an upcoming vacation or family reunion. You may be shocked at the number of social "excuses for throwing caution to the wind" you will find every single month. Most of us have at least one potential pitfall every single week!

- Be specific about what you are going to change. Set-ting goals that are specific and doable lead to success: setting unrealistic goals pave the way to failure and disappointment. If you are unsure of what is realistic, run your goal by a friend or family member that has good judgment and/or has knowledge in weight management. For example, if you tend to drink a lot of alcohol, it may not be realistic to set a goal of drinking only water at the next holiday. However, setting a goal of drinking two glasses of water in between every alcoholic beverage will certainly slow you down and help you stay hydrated.

- Don't stand near the food table! Fix yourself a plate and don't go back for seconds. (Good choices: olives, veggies, meat, fruit, whole grain crackers, and nuts.)

- Decide beforehand what you will have and tell someone who will hold you accountable (and write it down).

- For home celebrations, bring a healthy, delicious entrée to share so you are guaranteed at least one healthy food. For restaurant events, call and request a faxed copy of the menu or look at an online menu--you can make your meal decision before you go, without peer pressure.

- Find out your metabolic type® so that you know which foods to eat and which to avoid.

- Exercise before the party and schedule a workout the next day as well.

- Eat a snack before going to the party so that you aren't starving when you get there.

- Positive reinforcement: "Letting loose" is a frame of mind and a way of talking to yourself—if you tell yourself that you can have a great time without overindulging, you pave the road to success.

- Conscious eating--enjoy your food! Smell it, taste it, and chew it!

- Practice makes perfect–don't expect perfection on your first try. With each effort you make, your confidence will grow and making healthy decisions will get easier and easier.

Health Do's Checklist

- Eat a diet that makes you feel energetic, satisfied and clear-headed.

- Move your body every day.

- Drink half your body weight in ounces of filtered water daily MINIMUM!

- Eat foods that are free of pesticides, antibiotics, growth hormones, food coloring, high fructose corn syrup, agave (VERY processed), & artificial sweeteners as often as possible.

- Eat fats from many natural sources: coconut, grass-fed butter, flax, raw dairy, olive oil, raw nuts and seeds, healthy animals.

- Drink bone broth from a healthy animal every week to promote digestive health.

- Get some sunshine daily when weather permits.

- Sleep 7-8 hours every night.

- BONUS: Get tested for hidden stressors like food sensitivities, and imbalances with hormones, gut health, and neurotransmitters. Contact me through my website. www.choosinghealthnow.com for recommendations.

- Breathe!

Last Words of Advice

Opinions are like web pages--everyone's got one! People are all too quick to give out their opinion, even when they are in no way qualified to do so. Please, do me a favor: the next time someone tries to give you nutrition or exercise advice, ask them when they became a health professional. I know that sounds harsh, but we are inundated with faulty advice all day long and the consequences can be quite undermining. It probably isn't intentional, but friends and family members are doing you a huge disservice if their "helpful advice" prompts you to change your course of action from what a qualified health professional has recommended you do.

Sure, professionals can be wrong too. More than once have I read a book by a doctor and had it contradict years of schooling and personal experience. In this situation, I encourage you to use your instinct and seek a second opinion before blindly going along with their advice. In the end, your body will let you know when you are on the right track.

CHOOSING HEALTH

1. I choose to select a type of self-monitoring so that I can stay accountable weekly and make changes in my behavior before they become a problem. I choose to remind myself weekly of my commitment to my health.

2. I choose to self-monitor weekly and stay accountable--making changes in my behavior if I notice I am straying off-course. I will make healthy choices continuously, regardless of special occasions. I choose to remind myself weekly of my commitment to my health.

3. I choose to self-monitor daily and stay accountable--making changes in my behavior if I notice I am straying off-course. I

198

will make healthy choices continuously, regardless of special occasions. I choose to remind myself weekly of my commitment to my health.

Congratulations on completing your health makeover journey. You now have a complete set of tools to make and maintain healthy lifestyle changes. Refer to these tools often if you feel that you need motivation, reminders or ideas. Success takes ongoing effort and awareness. You have learned a great deal, but there is always more to learn. I am sure that you will make your own discoveries along the way: write them down and use them. You can never have too many tools. You will become an expert on your body.

Good luck to you on your ongoing journey of choosing health. :)

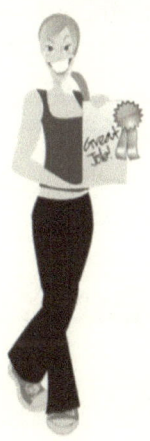

Thanks for reading Choosing Health!

If you found this information helpful, please leave a positive review on Amazon. It would help me out more than you can imagine, and I'd love to hear what you thought about the book!

Appendix A: Sample Menus

Sample Menu for Balanced Types

<u>Day One</u>

Breakfast: Mushroom & mozzarella omelette, Quinoa w/ butter, Fresh vegetable juice

Lunch: Chicken thigh, zucchini w/ garlic and butter, and arugula greens

Snack: Pecans, plain full-fat yogurt and raspberries

Dinner: Pot roast w/ onion, parsnip and Brussels sprouts, coconut oil

<u>Day Two</u>

Breakfast: Beef patty, Sautéed Kale, Sprouted gluten-free toast w/ Butter

Lunch: Turkey, lettuce and avocado salad w/ flax oil & balsamic dressing

Snack: Beef jerky & sliced cucumber

Dinner: Halibut w/ olive oil, herbs and lemon Roasted beets w/ ricotta, romaine salad

Day Three

Breakfast: Oatmeal, raw milk, chopped apple, cinnamon, soft boiled-egg

Lunch: Teriyaki salmon, bok choy and wild rice

Snack: Cottage cheese, strawberries and hazelnuts

Dinner: Lamb, onion and squash kabobs over kale

Day Four

Breakfast: Pork or chicken sausage, cooked in coconut oil, cantaloupe, coffee w/ cream

Lunch: Cottage cheese, walnuts, pineapple, green tea

Snack: Apple w/ goat cheese

Dinner: Cornish hen, quinoa, green beans and olive oil

Day Five

Breakfast: 1-2 organic chicken or turkey sausages, chopped pear, handful of almonds, 2 TBS feta or goat cheese

Lunch: Duck, broccoli and red potato w/ butter

Snack: Banana w/ peanut butter

Dinner: Shrimp, butter, kohlrabi and wild rice

Sample Menu for Carb Types

Day One

Breakfast: Ground chicken breast patty, sautéed spinach, 1 Slice sprouted gluten-free toast with butter

Lunch: Bean soup (white, pinto and navy) and green salad w/ beets and feta

Snack: Jicima and sunflower seeds

Dinner: Halibut, yam or sweet potato, drizzled in flax oil and almonds

Day Two

Breakfast: Oatmeal, blueberries, coconut oil

Lunch: Chicken breast, wild rice & broccoli drizzled in olive oil

Snack: Cottage cheese and cashews

Dinner: Black-eyed peas w/ bok choy & zucchini and parmesan cheese

Day Three

Breakfast: Sprouted gluten-free toast w/ banana and peanut butter

Lunch: Snapper w/ butter, tomato, peppers, and green salad

Snack: Full fat yogurt w/ almonds

Dinner: Turkey breast, mashed potato w/butter, and kale salad

Day Four

Breakfast: Poached egg, small amount of butter, and fresh vegetable juice

Lunch: Tomato and white bean soup w/ chicken stock, topped with sesame seeds

Snack: Beef jerky and Brazil nuts

Dinner: Cod, buttered Brussels sprouts, and spinach salad

Day Five

Breakfast: Mixed fruit, whipped ricotta cheese and Canadian bacon

Lunch: Ground chicken patty, lettuce, and potato fries baked in olive oil and rosemary

Snack: Hard boiled egg and sliced bell

Dinner: Cornish-hen, parsnips cooked in coconut oil, and butter lettuce topped with feta and pine nuts

Sample Menu for Protein Types

Day 1

Breakfast: Beef patty, sautéed spinach with butter, small serving of berries

Lunch: Skirt steak salad w/ spinach, celery & artichoke hearts, olive oil and herb dressing

Snack: Celery, peanut butter, turkey jerky

Dinner: Salmon, green beans drizzled in flax oil and pecans

Day 2

Breakfast: Ground pork, mushroom and cheddar omelette , small serving blueberries

Lunch: Chicken thigh, wild rice, asparagus drizzled in olive oil

Snack: Cottage cheese and walnuts

Dinner: Chicken thigh soup w/ carrots, celery, garlic, onion, herbs topped w/ parmesan cheese

Day 3

Breakfast: Smoked salmon & cream cheese on portobella mushroom

Lunch: Crab w/ butter, artichoke, and green salad

Snack: Full fat yogurt w/ macadamia nuts

Dinner: Lamb chop, mashed cauliflower w/ butter, and spinach salad

Day Four

Breakfast: Ground chicken thigh sausage on a bed of spinach, strawberries w/ brie cheese

Lunch: Lentil soup, cubed chicken thigh, and coconut oil

Snack: Beef jerky and Brazil nuts

Dinner: Buffalo steak, buttered carrots, and spinach

Day Five

Breakfast: Turkey thigh, w/ gouda and avocado over amaranth

Lunch: Ground beef patty, lettuce, and sweet potato fries baked in olive oil and rosemary

Snack: Hard boiled egg and pumpkin seeds

Dinner: Lobster w/ butter, corn and spinach topped with gorgonzola and hazelnuts

Appendix B: Recipes

Always use 100% grass-fed beef, free-range chicken and eggs, all natural pork, organic (preferably raw) dairy and organic produce.

<u>Main Courses</u>

Skirt Steak with Cauliflower

- 1 pound skirt steak
- Olive oil or butter
- 1 bunch cauliflower
- Grated Parmesan cheese

Use oil or butter in a large pan, put steak in the pan and turn on medium heat. Wash and cut up cauliflower into small pieces and steam with filtered water for 5 minutes. Cook steak for 3-5 minutes per side depending on how well done you like your meat. Once the cauliflower is soft enough, mash it with a potato masher or large fork, adding butter and Parmesan cheese to your liking.

Chili Con Carne

- 4 cups dry beans: mixture of black, pinto, and adzuki (soak over-night in filtered water and rinse thoroughly)
- 4 large tomatoes
- 2 pounds ground beef 2 jalapeno peppers
- 1 large green bell pepper
- 1tablespoons cayenne pepper 2 tablespoons chili powder
- 4 tablespoons organic hot sauce
- 1 teaspoon each of thyme and oregano

- Sea salt to taste

After soaking beans overnight and rinsing them completely, fill a pot with enough water so that it is 4 inches higher than the level of the beans. Add 2 teaspoons of sea salt and simmer with the lid on for 4 hours or until beans are soft. Next, chop up the bell pepper and tomatoes into small ½ inch pieces and dice the jalapeno peppers (seeds and all if you want it spicy). Add to the beans and crumble raw ground beef in as well. Add spices and simmer for another hour with the lid on, stirring occasionally.

Serve with cheddar cheese and sour cream. Makes over 20 servings.

Chicken & Veggie Soup

- 7-8 Chicken thighs with bones and skin (optional: cook whole chicken and strain out small bones at the end)
- 3 large carrots
- 3 large stalks of celery
- Filtered water
- Dried or fresh herbs
- Sea salt
- Optional: garlic and onions and almond meal to thicken and add delicious flavor!

The best soup stock is made with bones! Start a day ahead of time. Fill a large pot with filtered water and add chicken thighs. Cover and simmer all day, add 1/4 cup of apple cider vinegar. Chill overnight. Next day, cook on low heat for 5 more hours and then remove bones. Add fresh or dried herbs of your choice.

I like to make my soup with a tablespoon each of:

- Thyme, Rosemary, Oregano, and Sea salt

Add carrots and celery about an hour before serving.

Beef & Veggie Soup

- Beef bones (oxtail or marrow)
- 1-3 pounds of stew meat
- 3 large carrots
- 4 large stalks of celery
- Filtered water
- Dried or fresh herbs
- Sea salt
- Optional: garlic and onions and almond meal to thicken and add delicious flavor!

The best soup stock is made with bones! Start a day ahead of time and use either oxtail or marrow bones. Fill a large pot with filtered water and bones. Cover and simmer all day, add 1/4 cup of apple cider vinegar. Chill overnight. Next day, cook on low heat for 5 more hours and then remove bones. Add fresh or dried herbs of your choice.

I like to make my soup with a tablespoon each of:

- Thyme, Rosemary, Oregano, and Sea salt

Depending on how large your pot is, cook 1-3 pounds of cubed stew meat in a pan with a dash of red wine, celery and carrots. Add mixture to soup.

Coconut, Banana, Flax Smoothie

- ½ green banana (preferably frozen)
- 1-2 raw eggs
- ½ cup coconut milk
- ½ cup whole raw milk
- 2 tablespoons ground flax seeds
- Blend all contents in a blender thoroughly.

Coconut Fried Chicken

- 6 boneless, skinless chicken thighs
- Coconut oil
- 2-4 tablespoons

In a large skillet, melt coconut oil on low heat and then add chicken thighs. Turn heat up to medium and cover with a lid. Cook until thighs are done and add salt and pepper. Serves 3 with leftovers.

Coconut Chicken Curry

- 4 boneless skinless chicken thighs or breast 1 can coconut milk
- 4-5 sliced shiitake mushrooms
- 2 tablespoons each of garam masala and curry powder
- Sea salt
- Your choice of cooking greens (spinach, kale, chard, beet greens, collard greens, arugula)

Pour coconut milk into a medium pot. Add chicken, mushrooms, garam masala and curry powder. Simmer with lid on until chicken is cooked (about 15 minutes). Add cooking greens and cook for 5 minutes at the end OR eat the greens raw with chicken curry on top in a bowl. Serves 4.

Chicken Feta Burger

- 1-pound ground chicken thigh
- ¼ cup crumbled feta cheese
- 2 tablespoons dried basil
- Sea salt
- Coconut oil

Mix contents in a large bowl, form into patties and cook in coconut oil in a large covered skillet (8-10 minutes on medium heat). Serve over spinach or greens. Makes about 5 patties.

Salt and pepper to taste

Eggs with Spinach and Swiss cheese

- 1-2 eggs
- 1 cup fresh spinach
- 1-2 slices Swiss cheese
- Butter

Beat eggs in a bowl then pour into a small pan. Cook, covered, on low heat until eggs start to solidify. Toss in spinach and cheese and cover again. Stir as cheese starts to melt. Cook until done, then add salt and pepper. Serves 1.Optional: serve with a slice of Ezekiel toast and/or homemade pork sausage.

Pork Sausage

- 1-pound ground pork
- 1 teaspoon ground cumin 1 teaspoon dried basil
- ¼ teaspoon each of rosemary, thyme and oregano Sea salt

Mix together in a large bowl and make patties from mixture. I use a glass Tupperware bowl and keep the sausage mix in the refrigerator to cook as needed. Makes about 5 patties.

Southwest Chicken

- 4 chicken breasts, boneless skinless 1 Tomato
- 1 Jalapeno pepper
- 1 Red onion
- ½ cup cooked black beans
- ½ cup corn
- 1 teaspoon lime juice
- 1 teaspoon olive oil Pepper 2 gluten-free pitas or Paleo Wraps

Cook chicken breasts in a frying pan with a small amount of olive oil. Sprinkle them with pepper and lime juice. Cut up tomato, jalapeno (remove seeds), and red onion into small pieces and mix in black beans, corn, lime juice, oil, and some pepper. Mix it all up and then serve on the side of the chicken. Serve with a pita or wrap. Serves 4.

Mushroom Chicken

- 1 can of Amy's Organics cream of mushroom soup
- 2 boneless skinless chicken breasts
- ½ cup brown rice
- 1 large bunch broccoli
- ¼ cup sharp cheddar

Simmer chicken breasts in a small pot with the soup. Cook brown rice. Steam broccoli and sprinkle cheese on top. Serve chicken over rice and cover everything with a little soup. Serves 2.

Tempeh-Veggie Stir Fry

- 1 block organic tempeh
- 1 cups organic mixed cooking greens (beet, mustard, kale, chard)
- 3 cloves garlic
- ¼ cup gluten free teriyaki sauce
- 1 yellow onion
- ½ cup baby carrots cut in halves
- ½ cup mushrooms of choice
- 2 tablespoon olive or coconut oil
- ½ package Japanese style organic soba noodles
- 1 tablespoon sesame seeds

Boil 2 cups water in a pot. Crush garlic and let sit for 15 minutes. Put oil in wok under medium heat. Add onion, carrots, and greens, stirring occasionally until greens cook down. Put noodles in boiling water and cook until tender (3-5 minutes). Add mushrooms and tempeh (cut into cubes) and teriyaki sauce into stir fry and stir. Cook 2 minutes. Drain noodles and mix into stir fry. Top with sesame seeds. Serves 3.

Chicken Mandarin Orange Pasta

- 2 boneless skinless chicken breasts (free-range) cut into small cubes
- ¾ pound gluten-free rotelle pasta
- 1 can mandarin oranges, drained
- ¼ cup organic feta cheese
- 2 tablespoons olive oil
- 1 shallot
- 1 clove garlic
- Dash of Sea salt and black pepper to taste

Spray pan with olive oil. Sauté chicken on medium heat with chopped-up shallot and garlic. Boil water and add pasta (stir and reduce heat to medium-high). When pasta is cooked (but not too tender), drain and rinse with cool water and return to pot. Add chicken, onions, garlic and the drained orange slices. Mix in feta cheese, olive oil, and season with salt and pepper. Serve with your favorite veggie or salad.

Chicken & Vegetable Skewers

- 1 each: Free-range chicken breast, Red bell pepper, Red onion
- Optional: Mushrooms, pineapple, garlic, tofu, zucchini,
- eggplant

Chop ingredients into bite-sized pieces and slide onto skewer, alternating each ingredient. Brush with gluten-free teriyaki sauce. Grill until meat is fully cooked. 1 chicken breast serves 1 person.

Roasted Potato Medley

Cut sweet potatoes and red potatoes into bite-sized pieces and put into a large Tupperware bowl with a small amount of olive oil (1-2 tablespoons) and fresh rosemary. Put lid on and shake until potatoes are coated. Bake on a cookie sheet at 350 degrees until tender (approximately 30 minutes).

Rebecca's Meatloaf

- 3 lbs grass-fed ground beef
- Optional: 1/2 lb ground "pet food" (ground organ meats, they have to label it as pet food if the ground beef is under 70%)
- 1 organic carrot, chopped in 1/2-inch pieces
- 1/2 organic zucchini, chopped in 1/2-inch pieces
- 2 teaspoons each of ground onion, garlic
- 1 teaspoon each of sea salt, pepper, paprika, dried parsley, rosemary, and cumin

Pre-heat oven to 375. Mix everything in a large glass baking dish 8x10). and then press into a loaf. Bake for 45-60 mins. Serves 4 with leftovers.

Black Bean & Zucchini Squash

- 2-3 small zucchini squashes sliced
- ½ red onion diced
- ¼ cup sharp cheddar cheese
- 1 can organic black beans, rinsed (or even better--soak and cook your own)
- 1 can corn (or bag of frozen corn)
- 8 ounces of chunky salsa (try to choose lower-sodium salsa) 1 cup brown rice cooked with 2 tomatoes and 1/2 teaspoon cayenne pepper

Cook the rice using 1 tsp of olive oil in the boiling water. Add chopped tomatoes and cayenne pepper when halfway cooked. In a pan, use 1 tsp olive oil and pan-fry the squash for a few minutes, then add onion and cook until done. In a casserole dish, layer beans, rice, onion, squash, cheese, and salsa. Cover and bake for 20 mins at 400 degrees. Serves 4-5.

Baked Portabella Mushrooms

- 1 Portabello mushroom
- 1 teaspoon organic ghee, butter or coconut oil & lemon juice
- ½ teaspoon fresh lemon thyme, regular thyme, or rosemary
- 1 medium to large clove of garlic
- 1 tablespoon gluten-free bread crumbs

Crush garlic and set aside. Preheat oven to 350 degrees. Remove stem from mushroom and scoop out black gills and place under-side up in a baking dish. Melt butter and mix with lemon juice, thyme or rosemary and garlic. Scoop evenly over the mushroom and sprinkle with bread crumbs. Bake uncovered at 350 degrees for 10-15 minutes or until tender. Serves 1.

Spinach & Shrimp Pasta

- 1 16-ounce bag organic spinach
- 1 package Miracle Noodles (fettuccini)
- 1 ½ cups medium-sized shrimp (cooked)
- 2 cloves garlic
- 1 tablespoon fresh chives
- ¼ cup parmesan cheese
- 1 red bell pepper, chopped into 1-inch cubes
- Organic olive oil or butter as desired

Sauté garlic, spinach and bell peppers in a frying pan with 1 tablespoon olive oil, stirring often. When almost done, add shrimp. Take noodles out of package and rinse. Mix everything together, adding several more tablespoons of olive oil or butter and top with parmesan cheese. Serves 2-3.

Salads

Spinach Salad with Apples and Blue Cheese

- 1-pound spinach, washed, dried and torn into bite-sized pieces, stems discarded
- 1 Jonathan or Macintosh apples, washed, cored and cubed
- ¼ cup blue cheese crumbles

Mix ingredients together and dress with Conzorzio oil and vinegar dressing (organic and only 50 calories for 2 tablespoons). Serves 4.

Citrus Salad with Flax and Olive Oil Dressing

- 1 ruby red grapefruit 1 orange
- 12 large leaves red leaf lettuce, washed 1 avocado, cubed
- 2 tablespoons toasted sunflower seeds
- Dressing:
- 2 tablespoons extra virgin olive oil
- 1 tablespoon flaxseed oil
- 1 Tablespoon white balsamic vinegar 1 teaspoon lemon juice
- 2 tablespoons capers
- Salt and freshly ground black pepper to taste

Peel the grapefruit and orange and separate the segments, removing any seeds; cut the segments into chunks. (Retain the membrane for extra fiber and nutrients.) Combine in a large bowl. Tear the lettuce into bite-sized pieces. Add to the fruit mixture; stir in the avocado. In a small bowl, whisk together the olive oil, flaxseed oil, vinegar, lemon juice, and capers. Season with salt and pepper. Drizzle the dressing over the salad and toss lightly to combine. Transfer the salad to 6 plates and sprinkle 1 teaspoon of toasted sunflower seeds over each serving. (You can also use toasted pumpkin seeds.) Serves 6

Spinach Salad with Bacon & Blue Cheese

2-4 slices nitrite-free bacon
1-1½ cups raw spinach
¼ cup blue cheese crumbles Olive or flax oil

Cook bacon on stovetop or in oven (lay slices on cookie sheet, 350 degrees for 15 minutes for a whole package). Add bacon and blue cheese over spinach. Drizzle with either flax or olive oil and balsamic or apple cider vinegar if you desire.
Serves 1.

Hamburger Salad

- 1-pound ground beef
- 3 cups spinach or mixed greens
- Gorgonzola cheese
- Olive oil
- Balsamic vinegar
- Sea salt
- Black pepper
- Optional: garlic and onions, bell pepper

Form ground beef into palm-sized hamburger patties and cook in buttered pan on medium heat for 5 minutes (longer for well-done). If you are using the optional ingredients, throw them in while the hamburgers are cooking. On large plates, assembly greens. When burgers are done, put them on the greens and salt, pepper, cheese and oil/vinegar. Serves 3-5 depending on portion size.

Yummy Yogurt

- 1 cup plain organic yogurt
- 1 tsp vanilla extract
- ½ teaspoon cardamom
- 1/8 teaspoon coriander
- Vanilla stevia drops to taste (1-5 drops)

Mix together in a bowl. Serves 1.

Tropical Dessert

- ¾ cup plain organic yogurt
- ¼ cup fresh or frozen mango or papaya.

Top plain organic yogurt with fresh or frozen mango or papaya. Shredded coconut optional. Serves 1.

Baked Cinnamon Apples

- 4 organic apples (any kind)
- 4 tablespoons organic butter or ghee 1-4 teaspoons cinnamon
- 1 teaspoon coriander

Slice your favorite apples and arrange in a glass dish. Drizzle melted butter over apples. Spice with cinnamon (however much you like).

Bake at 400 degrees for 15-20 minutes until apples are tender. Optional: serve with fresh whipped cream OR over plain full-fat organic yogurt with or without crumbled graham crackers (make sure to buy a brand low in sugar and without partially hydrogenated oil). Crumbled walnuts on top is another delicious option. Serves 4.

Cardamom Banana Delight

- 1 large bananas (just ripened)
- 3-4 teaspoons of raw cocoa powder
- 1½ tablespoons cinnamon
- 2 teaspoons coriander
- 3 teaspoons cardamom
- 2 tablespoons butter

Slice bananas into pieces approximately ½ inch wide. In a large skillet, add butter and turn the heat on medium. Add banana slices, cocoa powder and spices and cook for 3-4 minutes, stirring so that the bananas get covered with spices and cocoa powder. Place into bowls and sprinkle more cardamom and/or cinnamon on top if you desire.

Optional: serve with fresh whipped cream OR over plain full-fat organic yogurt and sprinkle with raw walnuts. Serves 2.

Healthy Hot Chocolate

- 2 cups whole milk (or coconut or almond milk)
- 4 teaspoons raw cocoa powder
- 1 teaspoon cinnamon
- ½-1 tsp Lakanto
- Nutmeg

Heat milk in a pot on low heat until hot. Pour into 2 mugs. Add 2 teaspoons of cocoa powder, Lakanto and ½ teaspoon cinnamon and mix thoroughly. Grate fresh nutmeg on top and enjoy! If you want the cocoa sweeter, add more Lakanto. For a richer chocolate flavor, add more cocoa powder. Serves 2.

Spreads & Dips

Artichoke Pate

- ½ cup raw almonds
- Water for soaking
- 2 tablespoons raw pine nuts
- ¾ cup artichoke hearts, quartered
- 2 tablespoons water
- 2 teaspoons lemon juice
- 2 teaspoons garlic, minced
- ¼ teaspoon sea salt

Begin by placing the almonds in a small bowl covered with water. Then place in the refrigerator and leave them to soak overnight to loosen their skins. Remove the almonds from the water, squeeze each almond between your thumb and forefinger to remove the skin, place them on a towel, and set them aside to dry. Place the almonds and pine nuts in a blender or food processor, and finely grind for 1-2 minutes. Scrape down the sides of the container, add the remaining ingredients, and process for 1-2 minutes to form a smooth puree.

Taste and adjust seasonings as needed. Transfer the mixture to an airtight container and store in the refrigerator. Serve as a dip or spread for vegetables, crackers, or breads; as a sandwich filling; or to add flavor to sauces, dressings, salads, grains, or other side dishes.
Yield: 1 ¼ Cups.

Black Bean Hummus

- 1 can black beans, drained (15 ounces)
- ¼ cup tahini
- 1 tablespoon garlic, minced
- 1 tablespoon olive oil
- ¼ tablespoon lime juice
- ½ teaspoon cumin
- ½ teaspoon cayenne pepper

In a food processor, process all ingredients until smooth and creamy. If it is too thick, add half a teaspoon olive oil and a half teaspoon lime juice. Serve immediately or store in refrigerator in airtight container.
Yields about 1 cup.

Appendix C: References

The American heritage® dictionary of the english language, fourth edition (2007, October 28). Diet. (n.d.). Retrieved October 28, 2007, from Answers.com website: http://www.answers.com/topic/dieting

AskDrSears.com (2006). *The joy of soy.* Retrieved from http://www.askdrsears.com/html/4/T044700.asp

Aukerman, G. (2007). *Understanding omega-3 and omega-6,* Retrieved November 25, 2007, from NetWellness website: http://www.netwellness.org /healthtopics/alternative/omega3. cfm

Bailey, C. (1994). *Smart exercise.* New York: Houghton Mifflin.

Batmanghelidj, F. (2003). *You're not sick, you're thirsty!* New York: Warner Books.

Bauer, K. & Sokolik, C. (2002). *Nutritional counseling.* Belmont: Wadsworth/Thomson Learning.

Bland, J. et al. (1999). *Clinical nutrition: A functional approach.* Gig Harbor: Institute for Functional Medicine.

Dr. Sandra Cabot's Liver Doctor. (2007, November 3). *Toxins in food and in the environment.* Retrieved from http://www.liver-doctor.com/index.php?page=liver-problems&subpage=toxins

Calorie Control Council. (2007, November 24). *Reduced-calorie sweeteners: Tagatose.* Retrieved from Caloriecontrol.org website: http://www.caloriecontrol.org/tagatose.html

Cabot, S. (2006). *The liver cleansing diet.* Glendale: S.C.B.

International.

Castner, K. (2001). *Metabolism*. San Diego: American Council on Exercise.

Chek, P. (2004). How to eat, move, and be healthy. San Diego:

C.H.E.K. Institute

Cichoke, A. (2000). *Enzymes and enzyme therapy*. Chicago: Keats.

Crohn's.net (no date provided). *Essential fatty acids*. Retrieved on November 25, 2007 from http://www.crohns.net/Miva/education/aboutEFAs.shtml

Dodd, S. (2005). *Mom Looks Great*. Charleston: BookSurge.

Egoscue, P. & Gittines, R. (1998). *Pain free*. New York: Bantom Books.

Erasmus, U. (2003). *Fats that heal, fats that kill*. Burnaby: Alive Books.

Fallon, S. & Enig, M. (1995, September 27). *The ploy of soy*.

Retrieved December 19, 2009 from Weston A. Price Foundation website: http://www.westonaprice.org/The-Ploy-of-Soy.html

Fallon, S. and Enig, M. (2002, September 8). *Teens before their time*.

Retrieved December 15, 2007 from Weston A. Price Foundation website: http://www.westonaprice.org/soy/teensbe-foretime.html

Food Navigator (2004, May 29). *Low-cal sweetener has low-GI, new study*. Retrieved from http://www.foodnavigator.com/ Financial-Industry/Low-cal-sweetener-has-low-GI-new-study

Feskanich, D., Willett, W.C., Stampfer, MJ., & Colditz, GA., (1996). *Protein consumption and bone fractures in women.*

Department of Nutrition, Harvard School of Public Health 143(5), 472-9. Retrieved from http://aje.oxfordjournals.org/cgi/reprint/143/5/472.pdf

Fife, B. (2001). *The detox book.* Colorado Springs: Piccadilly Books.

Fitzpatrick, M. (2009, February 27). *Soy isoflavones: Panacea or poison?*

Retrieved December 24, 2009 from Weston A. Price

Happy Stomach (no date provided). *All about stevia.* Retrieved November 24, 2007 from http://www.happystomach. com/stevia.htm

Harvard School of Public Health. (2010). *Protein: Moving closer to center stage.* Retrieved from http://www.hsph.harvard. edu/nutritionsource/protein.html

Heaney, R. (2002). Protein and calcium: Antagonists or synergists?

American Journal of Clinical Nutrition, 75(4), 609-610. http://www.ajcn.org/

Hidgon, J. (2006, January). *Soy isoflavones.* Retrieved December 19, 2007 from Linus Pauling Micronutrient Center for Optimum Health website: http://lpi.oregonstate.edu/infocenter/phytochemicals/soyiso/#soy_formula

Holford, P. (2000). *The optimum nutrition bible.* Freedom: The Crossing Press.

Karpay, E. (2000) *The everything total fitness book.* Holbrook: Adams Media Corporation.

Kendrick, M. (2008) *The great cholesterol con.* London: John Blake.

Kirkland, J. & T. (2002). *Sugar-free cooking with stevia.* Arlington: Crystal Health Publishing.

Kirschenbaum, D. (2000).*The 9 truths about weight loss.* New York: Henry Holt and Company.

Leduc, M. (2002). *Is soy healthy?* Retrieved January 20, 2008 from Healing Daily website: http://www.healingdaily.com/detox-ification- diet/soy.htm

Liebman, B. (1997, June). *Where's the ground beef labeling?* Retrieved January 20, 2008 from Nutrition Action Healthletter website: http://www.cspinet.net/nah/junebeef.htm

MacArthur , J. (2004, April 28). *Soy and the brain.* Retrieved December 14, 2007 from Weston A. Price Foundation website: http://www.westonaprice.org/soy/soyandbrain.html

May, J. (no date provided). *Stevia-sweetener of choice for future generations.* Retrieved November 18, 2007 from Healthy. Net website: http://www.healthy.net/scr/article.asp?id=2413

The Mayo Clinic (2007, November 14). *Wheat allergy.* Retrieved from http://www.mayoclinic.com/health/wheat-allergy/ DS01002/DSECTION=1

Mangels, R. (2006). *Expert panel evaluates soy safety.* Vegetarian Journal. Retrieved from http://findarticles.com/p/articles/ mi_m0FDE/is_4_25 /ai_n16834303

Merritt, R., Henkel, J. and Jenks, H. (2004). *Soy: Health claims for soy protein, Questions about other components.* Retrieved December 20, 2007 from FDA website: http://www.fda. gov/fdac/features/2000/300_soy.html

Merritt, R.J. & Jenks, B.H. (2004). Safety of Soy-based Infant Formulas Containing Isoflavones: The Clinical Evidence. *The American Journal of Nutritional Sciences*. 134(5). doi:134:1220S-1224S

Myers, T. (2001). *Anatomy trains.* Philadelphia: Churchill Livingstone.

Nordqvist, C. (2004, May 27). *What is the vegetarian diet?*

What are the benefits of a vegetarians diet? Retrieved December 16, 2007 from Medical News Today website: http://www.medicalnewstoday.com/articles/8749.php

Organic Valley Pastures. (2007, October 29). *Frequently asked questions.* Retrieved October 29, 2007, from Organic Valley Pastures website: http://www.organicpastures.com/faq.html

The oxford companion to the body. (2007, October 28). *Diet. (n.d.).* Retrieved October 28, 2007 from Answers.com web site: http://www.answers.com/topic/dieting

Pentz, J. (2006, October). Reading underneath the label, understanding food labeling regulations. *ACE Certified News,* 30-33.

Pope, R.P., Herbert, R.D., Kirwan, J.D., Graham, B.J. (2000). A Randomized Trial of Pre-exercise Stretching for Prevention of Lower-limb Injury. *Medicine & Science in Sports & Exercise*, 32(2).

Retrieved from-www.ncbi.nlm.nih.gov/ pubmed/10694106

Price, W. (1939). *Nutrition and physical degeneration.* La Mesa: Price-Pottenger Nutrition Foundation.

Quinn, E. (2008, January 18). Preventing overtraining-when less is more.

Retrieved December 9, 2007 from About.com website: http://sportsmedicine.about.com/cs/overtraining/a/ aa062499a.htm

Quorn Foods Inc. (2006) *What is quorn?* Retrieved December 18, 2007 from www.quorn.us/cmpage.aspx?pageid=372

Raskin, D. (2006) *The everything easy fitness book*. Holbrook: Adams Media Corporation.

Roizen, Michael F. and Oz, Mehmet C. (2006). *You on a diet.* New York: Free Press.

Schwarzbein, D. (2005).The Schwartzbein principle: The program.

Deerfield Beach: Health Communications, Inc.

Sharkey, B. (2002). *Fitness & health*. Champaign: Human Kinetics.

Steinman, H. (2002, May). *Milk allergy and lactose intolerance*, Retrieved November 14, 2007 from Science in Africa website: www.scienceinafrica.co.za/2002/may/milk.htm

Swithers, S., & Davidson, T. (2008). A Role for Sweet Taste: Calorie Predictive Relations in Energy Regulations by Rats. *Behavioral Neuroscience*, 122(1), 161-173. Retrieved from www.ncbi.nlm.nih.gov/pubmed/18298259

Taubes, G. (2008). *Good calories, bad calories*. New York: Anchor Books.

U.S. Food and Drug Administration, Center for Food Safety and Applied Nutrition. (2000). *How to understand and use the nutrition facts panel*. Retrieved from www.cfsan.fda. gov/~dms/foodlab.html#twoparts

U.S. Department of Agriculture, Agricultural Research Service.

(2005). *Get the skinny on lean beef.* Retrieved January 20, 2008 from About.com website: http://lowfatcooking.about.com/gi/dynamic/offsite.htm?zi=1/XJ&sdn=lowfatcooking&cdn=food&tm=21&f=10&su=p674.2.400.ip_p284.8.150.ip_&tt=12&bt=1&bts=1&zu=http%3A//www.beefitswhatsfordinner.com/nutrition/leancuts.asp

The Vegetarian Society (2007). *Protein.* http://www.vegsoc. Org http://www.vegsoc.org/info/protein.html

WebMD (2007, November 12). *Allergies: Problem foods: Is it an allergy or an intolerance?* Retrieved from http://www.webmd.com/allergies/guide/foods- allergy-intolerance

Weston A. Price Foundation (2007). *Myths & truths about soy.*

Retrieved from http://www.whale.to/a/soy2.html

Wolcott, W. & Fahey, T. (2000). *The metabolic typing diet.* New York: Broadway Books.

Wood, D. (2005). *Fluoride and your bones: A mixed bag.* Retrieved December 24, 2007 from NYU Langone Medical Center website: http://www.med.nyu.edu/patientcare/library/article.html?ChunkIID=14731

The World's Healthiest Foods. (2007, December 5). *Protein.*

Retrieved from http://www.whfoods.com/genpage.php?tname=nutrient&dbid=92

Whitney, E. & Rolfes, S. (2002). *Understanding nutrition.* Belmont: Wadsworth/Thomson Learning.

Wiley, R. (1989). *BioBalance.* Orem: Essential Science Publishing.

About the Author

Rebecca Hazelton is a licensed Nutritionist, Functional Diagnostic Nutrition Practitioner, and HeartMath Stress Resilience Coach.

She works with people across the globe whose health symptoms are forcing them to stop living life fully. She helps them to regain their health so they can feel great and free to enjoy life again.

She has authored 2 books Choosing Health: A One-Size-Doesn't-Fit-All Guide to Diet, Exercise & Motivation

And Pleasure Meditation: Your Guide to Joyful Stress Reduction.

Go to choosinghealthnow.com to check out her books, blog, previous interviews, and Unstoppable Health coaching programs.

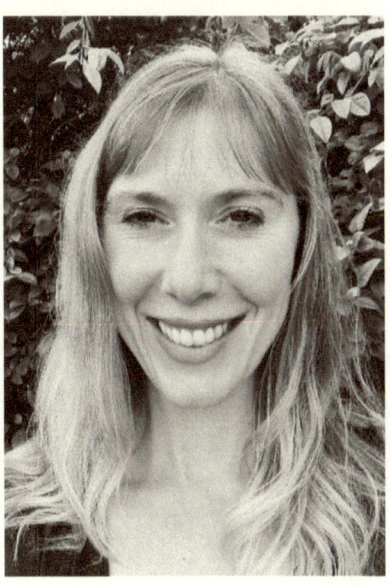